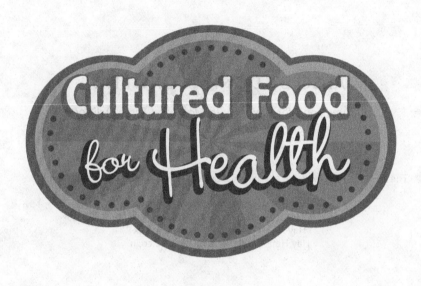

ALSO BY DONNA SCHWENK

Cultured Food for Life: How to Make and Serve Delicious
Probiotic Foods for Better Health and Wellness

The above book is available at your local bookstore, or may be ordered by visiting:

Hay House USA: www.hayhouse.com®
Hay House Australia: www.hayhouse.com.au
Hay House UK: www.hayhouse.co.uk
Hay House India: www.hayhouse.co.in

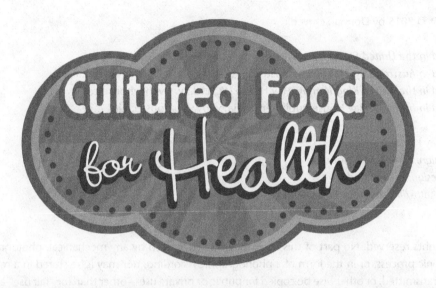

A Guide to Healing Yourself with Probiotic Foods

DONNA SCHWENK

HAY HOUSE, INC.
Carlsbad, California • New York City
London • Sydney • New Delhi

Published in the United States by: Hay House, Inc.: www.hayhouse.com®
Published in Australia by: Hay House Australia Pty. Ltd.: www.hayhouse.com.au
Published in the United Kingdom by: Hay House UK, Ltd.: www.hayhouse.co.uk
Published in India by: Hay House Publishers India: www.hayhouse.co.in

Indexer: Jay Kreider
Cover design: Amy Rose Grigoriou
Interior design: Riann Bender
Interior photos/illustrations: Maci Dierking

Cataloging-in-Publication Data is on file with the Library of Congress

Tradepaper ISBN: 978-1-4019-7242-4

1st edition, October 2015

Printed in the United States of America

To my husband, Ron, who tells me again and again:
"A rising tide lifts all boats."

CONTENTS

CONTENTS

YOUR CULTURED FOOD GUIDE

Dramatically improve your health by eating foods filled with dynamic probiotics that supercharge your body! Join Donna Schwenk at www.culturedfoodlife.com—a special place where you can go to find information and inspiration. Learn not only how to make cultured foods but also how to make them in ways that your entire family will love. There are numerous resources to help you on this new and exciting journey. Check out just a few:

- **Free recipes, articles, and videos**—plus a free *Getting Started Guide* e-book—to help you begin your journey.

- **Hundreds of photos,** including images of most of the foods in this book.

- **Online store** with links to products and ingredients mentioned in this book—and that Donna uses every day when making cultured foods. Just visit www.culturedfoodlife.com/store.

- **Up-to-date, worldwide information** on where to get culturing products and ingredients, including Cutting Edge starter culture. Go to www .culturedfoodlife.com/worldwide to learn more.

- **A community of enthusiasts** who have shared dozens of inspiring testimonials about how cultured foods changed their lives. These are the stories that keep Donna going day after day.

- **Biotic Pro membership** that gives you access to premium content, including exclusive online recipes and hours of quality videos culled from Donna's classes and her home-cooking adventures—there's even one about making cultured foods on a boat. Plus, you can catch **"Donna's Road Map,"** her series of mini videos that answer all your questions about creating and enjoying cultured foods. Check out www.culturedfoodlife.com /members.

- **Membership Forum**, a place (to which, as a Biotic Pro, you'll have access) where you can ask questions, share your stories, and get help with anything and everything related to cultured foods.

To all of you who've avoided cultured foods, thinking that they're daunting and difficult, visit www.culturedfoodlife.com to find out just how simple it is to incorporate these foods into your life and to learn how easy they are to prepare.

INTRODUCTION

*"You take people, you put them on a journey, you give
them peril, you find out who they really are."*

—Joss Whedon

Why did you pick up this book, and how did you find it?

I don't believe in coincidences. I believe that we are drawn to the things we need whether we know it or not. My guess is that you're not feeling well. That you've been searching for something that will help you take care of those digestive problems or those hay fever symptoms. That you're looking for a natural way to handle your diabetes or high blood pressure. And let me say, you've been drawn to the right place.

This is exactly what happened to me 13 years ago, when, sick and depressed, I happened upon a quote by Hippocrates, the father of Western medicine, that shook me to my core:

"All disease begins in the gut."

What did this mean? At the time I had no idea, but I wanted to find out. In fact, it became my mission. And that's when I discovered cultured foods—specifically kefir, kombucha, and cultured vegetables. I now refer to these three things as the Trilogy, a healing powerhouse of foods.

When I started eating cultured foods, every ailment I had went away. I watched as these foods healed my tiny baby. Then they healed my teenager from irritable bowel syndrome. I was astounded as they worked miracles in my friends and their children. Problems like ulcers, asthma, and digestive issues went away completely. How could something so simple change everybody?

What I learned is that eating cultured foods floods your body with billions of good bacteria that help balance your gut, which allows your body to heal itself. And this is exactly what I want for you.

In these pages, I lay out both the science behind how these foods work and information about how to incorporate them into your own life. I'll show you, step by step, how to make each one and give you some of my favorite recipes, plus hints and tips about how to bring them into your daily routine. I've also laid out a 21-day plan that takes you by the hand and explains in very clear terms what to do each day in an effort to eat all three foods.

You may be hesitant to try cultured foods at first, but I hope you will let me help you. We'll walk this road together. I think it's time; don't you? Grab a cup of tea and a comfy spot and let's begin together, just you and me.

I hope we can have an epidemic of wellness, and I hope I can help you believe in your own wellness. It is the sweetest way to live your life.

PART I

Fermenting Health

CHAPTER 1

The Hundred Trillion Friends You Didn't Know You Had

*Struggles will always reveal true friends—
and perhaps friends you never knew you had.*

I know this may be hard to believe, but your body is constantly remaking itself. Your lungs are only two to three weeks old and the cells in them are constantly renewing themselves. Your intestines are being replaced every two to three days. The surface layer of your skin is new every two to three weeks, and your liver is new every five months. It may sound crazy, but you can take 70 percent of someone's liver away in an operation and about 90 percent will grow back in two months.

When I first heard this, I didn't really believe it. But now I've experienced firsthand how self-healing and amazing the human body can be—as long as you supply it with what it needs to thrive.

If you have heard my story before, you know that I was a new mom at 41 years old with diabetes, high blood pressure, and a four-pound preemie who was delivered seven and a half weeks early to save my life. Thankfully the story didn't end there. Instead, it was a wake-up call. I *had* to find a way to get healthy so my baby and the rest of my family wouldn't have to live without me. I felt desperate, so I went on a search for help.

In this search, I was drawn to probiotic foods, which contain live, good-for-you bacteria—just as you were drawn to this book. Filled with an unquenchable yearning, I started to bring them into my life. I didn't know what they would do, but I craved them. And what I found was that they reversed the symptoms and life-threatening warning signs in my own life—and they made my young infant thrive like never before. How could these special foods have such an impact on my tiny baby and me?

This question set me on a new path of research and learning, while its subject—cultured foods—helped me overcome the despair I was feeling. My sadness turned to joy, and every single area of my life began to change. I discovered so many things about my body, such as the hundred trillion best friends I didn't even know I had.

Making Friends with Bacteria

The number of bacteria in your body is astounding—somewhere around ten times the number of cells you have. And they're not just in you; they're everywhere. They come in all shapes: some look like rods, others are spherical or spirals. And they're all too tiny to see with the naked eye. Sadly, most of the news we hear about bacteria is bad—they create illness and disease, and sometimes they can even kill you. These stories have led to an extreme uptick in the use of antibiotics and antibacterial soaps. And then the prevalence of these products reinforces the idea that bacteria are bad. But the majority of the bacteria in your body are actually good for you. It's sad—we have not simply overlooked their importance; we have demonized them. We have actually forgotten that bacteria are largely responsible for keeping us well each and every day.

Good bacteria are a mighty force inside of you, but these microbes must strengthen and increase in number in order to keep you healthy. When there are enough organisms of certain species, they form an army to do their jobs—developing the immune system, breaking down foods, fighting bad bacteria, and so much more. They do things that you need for health but that can't be done by any other system in the body. This can best be illustrated in the stomach of a cow. Cows can't break down the cellulose in plants on their own, but they need to in order to get nutrients from it. So bacteria do it for them, breaking the food into simple sugars that the cows' bodies can use. This gives them all the energy they need to thrive. Bacteria do this for us, too. They help in the synthesis of vitamins K, B1, B2, B3, B6, and B12; folic acid; pantothenic acid; and some amino acids. They also help us absorb minerals, break down toxins, and produce a number of enzymes that break down proteins, carbohydrates, fiber, and fats.

You are a hundred trillion bacteria. They are in you, on you, and all around you. And if you tend to them, they can do amazing things for you. However, if you kill the bad bacteria without building up the good ones, it leaves you in a precarious position as the bad bacteria can mutate and get stronger. Building up the good bacteria, inside you and all around you, is the key to living a healthy life. When good bacteria dominate, you're living in a natural balance and everyone thrives.

The Amazing Power of the Invisible

You know how I just mentioned that our bodies remake themselves? Bacteria are a huge part of this process. The beneficial bacteria within us break down our food and transform it into vitamins, minerals, and other nutrients that nourish and create the bodies we live in. And it all starts at birth.

When you were in your mother's womb, you were in a sterile environment; you had no bacteria. But when you passed through the birth canal or entered the world through a cesarean section, you were infused with bacteria from everywhere—your mother, your father, the doctors, the nurses, the environment—pretty much anyone and anything you came in contact with affected the bacteria in your system. This is important because it laid the foundation of your inner world. As you entered this world, you basically became bacteria.

But this is the really exciting part: once you created this base of bacteria, your bacteria started talking to your cells about all aspects of your life and health. They helped train your immune system to recognize the bad, disease-producing bacteria so it could protect you. They helped your body produce the vitamin K that's necessary for normal blood clotting and for bone health.

As your body laid this foundation of microflora, bacteria talked to special markers in your gut to determine how things were going to run. They talked to these markers by attaching to them, and if the markers got the types of bacteria they needed, then everything ran smoothly. But if they didn't, they became damaged. All of this work the bacteria did at the beginning of your life continues to this day, which means that you can take advantage of this in order to heal many ailments you may have.

Recently, researchers at New York University Medical Center made some exciting discoveries regarding food allergies and intestinal bacteria. Not only did they discover why children develop food allergies, but they also found a way to solve the problem. The study, which was published in the *Proceedings of the National Academy of Sciences*, found that young children who were given too many antibiotics early on were at greater risk of developing food allergies. The researchers identified naturally occurring bacteria in the human gut that keep people from developing food allergies; if these bacteria were killed by antibiotics early in life, children became more susceptible to food allergies later on.

The scientists tested this theory by feeding antibiotics to young mice and found they were more likely to develop a peanut sensitivity than the control group was. When the young mice were then given the good bacterium *Clostridium*, like magic their allergic reactions vanished.[1]

Bacteria aren't responsible only for a healthy body, either—having a healthy gut also leads to a healthier emotional state. Before I found cultured foods, I was a different person— physically and emotionally. As a young woman, and all the way into my late 30s, I would get upset easily. I didn't smile often and simply wasn't that happy. I am sad to say that I often felt grouchy and snapped at my kids. But when I started to eat cultured foods, everything changed. The summer I started to clean up my diet, I also started to realize that I wasn't getting overly cross with my kids. I began to wonder how food, especially cultured food, could change someone's state of being so much. Since this realization, I've come upon research that helps me understand what happened in my life.

An article published in *Natural News* talks about a study out of Oxford University in the U.K. led by Dr. Drew Ramsey. The article discusses Dr. Ramsey's findings: "Nutrient deficiency is a major cause of behavioral abnormalities. Without the proper nutrients . . . the body cannot produce the appropriate chemicals and hormones required for clear thinking and healthy mood, which in turn can lead to irrational and even dangerous behaviors."

The study he conducted, in an attempt to see just how diet affects mood and behavior, was done with prison inmates split into two groups: the first was given vitamin supplements and the second was given a diet of junk food. What he found is that the people in the first group became much calmer and less aggressive.

The article also quoted a nutritionist named Nicolette Pace, who said, "Deficiencies in nutrients, magnesium or manganese, vitamin C, or some B vitamins may make a person hyperactive towards a stressor, a short fuse so to speak." Carbohydrates, she continued, "don't give your body what you need to cope with day-to-day stresses."[2] This means that anything you can do to help your body absorb more nutrients, such as get more healthy bacteria in your gut, will help your emotional state.

A compelling link between gut health and mental health was also directly established by a study led by John Cryan, a neuroscientist in Ireland. In his study, anxious mice that were dosed with the probiotic bacterium *Lactobacillus rhamnosus* showed lower levels of anxiety, decreased stress hormones, and even an increase in brain receptors for a neurotransmitter that is vital in curbing worry, anxiety, and fear.[3] Why would this happen? One reason is that 90 percent of the body's total serotonin—the feel-good chemical that leads to happiness and a sense of well-being—is produced in the digestive tract. Only 5 percent is produced in the brain. So creating a healthy digestive tract is essential for producing the chemicals that lead to a good mood. And creating a healthy digestive tract is all about what you're putting in your body.

CREATING DIGESTIVE HEALTH

Our diets and food sources have changed dramatically in the past 50 years. We have traded whole, unprocessed foods for convenience in a can or box. We want it to be cheap, fast, and readily available. In addition, many of our fruits, vegetables, nuts, and seeds are being genetically modified and sprayed with pesticides like never before. I wish the person I am now could talk to the young woman I was when I was experiencing such terrible health problems. That way I could tell her how important healthy eating is.

I grew up on a typical processed-food diet in an era when convenience became the most important factor in meal preparation. Cereal, TV dinners, and spaghetti in a can were superfast, and they appealed to kids and busy moms alike. My mom would cook unprocessed meals, too, but we became accustomed to the fast foods and wanted them more than the real thing. Besides, real, whole food wasn't as cool as the stuff promoted on TV. Consequently I suffered, and so did my children. And not just my children. Kids around the world are getting diseases that used to crop up only in later adulthood, and it's happening at an alarming rate. Just as I have seen in my own life, much of it seems to stem from diet and lifestyle choices.

We can see the connection between diet and health in a decadelong nutrition study done by Francis M. Pottenger, Jr., M.D., on multiple generations of cats. There were two groups of cats: The first group was fed a diet composed of raw meat, cod-liver oil, and raw dairy. (Contrary to popular belief, raw milk has good bacteria in it.) The second group was fed a diet of cooked meat and pasteurized milk plus cod-liver oil. So what happened?

The cats in the first group remained healthy and gave birth to healthy kittens with each generation. All vitamins and minerals were present in normal amounts in their blood. Their nervous systems functioned normally, and their coordination was perfect. They were very resistant to infections. Their mental state was stable and friendly, and you could play with them.

The second group gave birth to healthy babies in the first generation, but the offspring developed diseases and illnesses near the end of their lives. The onset of illness came in midlife in the second generation of offspring. The third generation began manifesting signs of poor health near the beginning of their lives, and many died before six months of age. Ailments affecting the heart, thyroid, bladder, nervous system, ovaries and testes, and liver were all present, along with increasingly poor eyesight (nearsightedness or farsightedness), meningitis, paralysis, inflammation, uterine congestion, and infection and atrophy of various organs.

What's more, with each new generation, the cats became more unpredictable, more irritable, less playful, and more prone to biting and scratching. The males became docile, experiencing a drop in libido and sexual interest, while the females became aggressive. They also began to miscarry in the first generation, and about 70 percent of the offspring in the second generation miscarried. In all cases the delivery was difficult, and sometimes the females died giving birth. Sadly, there was no fourth generation of these cats—not one cat in the third generation could give birth to healthy offspring. Either the third-generation parents were sterile or the fourth-generation cats died before birth.

I realize we aren't cats, but there are some similar things happening at this time in so many people's lives. The rates of infertility and autoimmune diseases are rising significantly. But all this can change if we simply change our diets. And this is where cultured foods come in.

These foods have so much beneficial bacteria that consuming them on a regular basis not only makes you feel better but also builds your body's ability to fight and cure illness. Our bodies were designed to heal themselves with extraordinary efficiency. They have a divine intelligence, and once you start to pay attention to the foods you eat and how they affect you, you will begin to work with your body and become the master of your destiny. You can heal yourself—if you simply give your body what it needs.

CHAPTER 2

The Trilogy

Change yourself from the inside out.

I want to tell you all about the health benefits of the Trilogy. But first, I need to introduce you to exactly what it is.

The Trilogy is made up of three magical, powerful cultured foods that I consume every day without fail. They are kefir, kombucha, and cultured vegetables. They are my best friends and my secret weapons. And they have changed my life because they not only are delicious but also have the extraordinary ability to speak to the cells of my body, changing it from the inside out. These three foods have made me healthier and happier than I can express. And they can do the same for you. You simply have to bring them into your life. I'll describe exactly how to do this later in the book, but for now, you just need to know that it is possible to take your average, run-of-the-mill food or drink and make it into a healing powerhouse by using a simple process called culturing.

The basic idea of culturing is this: you combine a food or beverage with a starter culture, which is a collection of live, healthy bacteria and yeasts, and then you set the conditions to make those bacteria and yeasts grow and thrive. These good microbes multiply so much that they overpower any bad microbes, which both preserves your food and makes it super rich in probiotics. This is why cultured foods and drinks are so powerful.

There are a couple of things to keep in mind when looking for the utmost healing from consuming cultured foods. The first is that you need to note the *and* of the Trilogy. It's kefir, kombucha, *and* cultured vegetables. While each of these foods promotes health on its own, it's really the combination of all three that has amazing healing powers. Over the years I've helped hundreds of people incorporate cultured foods into their lives, and I've seen extraordinary changes in their health. Early in my work, I began to notice the importance of the *and.* When people consumed one part of the Trilogy they would get better, but when they consumed all three they would thrive! Some of these changes seemed utterly miraculous. And as I learned more, what I found out is that each food in the Trilogy contains a different set of bacteria and yeasts that we need in order to flourish. Kefir, kombucha, and cultured vegetables are all chock-full of good bacteria, but they're all different, so to get the biggest effect you need all three.

The second thing to remember is that the homemade versions of these foods are much stronger and provide more benefits than the store-bought versions. Trying the options at your local market is an easy way to begin, but I highly recommend that you make and eat your own.

Each one of these foods trained me to eat it. One by one, kefir, kombucha, and cultured veggies got my attention. Some of the healing effects were dramatic, and others were more subtle, growing over time. This gave me the opportunity to find out just what they could do to support me and bring balance to my life. We learn best by life experience. Feeling better and seeing ourselves change and heal are more convincing than anything else. So let me introduce you to my three good friends!

KEFIR

Kefir was the first food in the Trilogy that I tried, and I think it's a great place to start. It's the most familiar feeling of the cultured foods, plus it's quick and easy to make. You can have homemade kefir in as little as 24 hours!

This cultured milk product, which can be made with any kind of milk—cow, goat, coconut, almond—is a cousin of yogurt. It's thinner and often a little bubbly, and it's fantastically energizing to drink. Kefir has much more powerful probiotic effects than yogurt because homemade kefir has 30 to 56 different strains of bacteria, as opposed to the 7 to 10 found in yogurt. Yogurt keeps the stomach happy, but only for a day or so. Kefir, on the other hand, with its stronger strains of bacteria, helps recolonize the good flora in your gut, keeping your belly happy in the long term. Kefir's special microbes will make your body their home and keep things in balance.

Another difference between yogurt and kefir is that the bacteria in kefir are naturally occurring. Today most of the yogurts we consume are pasteurized, which means that heat is used to kill off bacteria before good microbes are added back in. This is great in terms of killing bad bacteria, but it also kills a lot of enzymes and helpful bacteria, and when the good bacteria are reintroduced, they aren't added in nearly as high a concentration. Kefir is never heated, so it keeps all the healthy nutrients and good flora it began with. It is made in the old tradition of fermentation, which means that the only heat used is generated by the microbes themselves. Before refrigerators, fermentation was how people kept their food from spoiling—the healthy bacteria multiplied and preserved the food, keeping it safe.

Kefir is a powerhouse of not only good bacteria but probiotic yeast as well, yet another ally in your fight for a balanced gut. Yeast is what makes kefir bubbly—the reason it is often referred to as "the champagne of yogurt."

One serving of kefir has as much as 35 percent of the daily recommended allowance of protein, lots of vitamins A, B, C, and K, and phosphorus. It is loaded with enzymes, which help you get more nutrients from your food, and is virtually sugar- and lactose-free because the bacteria in it has eaten both of those things.

Another great thing about kefir is that it requires very little effort on the part of the body to extract nutrition from it. Digestion requires a large amount of the body's energy, but because kefir is partly digested (that's what fermentation is), the body can easily access its goodness.

I can't say enough about all the health benefits of kefir. While I'll go deeper into the science of cultured foods in Chapter 4, just know that when you consume kefir, it will help your digestion, reduce inflammation, make elimination a breeze, and so much more. I had one grateful mom tell me that when she started to give her child kefir, it killed the *Helicobacter pylori* (the bacterium that causes ulcers) in her stomach and healed her daughter's multiple ulcers when nothing else would. These harmful bacteria could not survive when the powerful good bacteria in kefir dominated her gut.

KOMBUCHA

In simple terms, kombucha is a bubbly, fermented tea made by combining tea, sugar, and a kombucha starter culture of bacteria and yeast called a SCOBY. The taste is rather tart, and, depending on what kind of tea you use, it can resemble anything from apple cider to champagne. I love it! There is nothing else like it.

NOTED HEALTH BENEFITS OF KEFIR

- Eliminates constipation
- Reduces or eliminates allergies
- Enhances digestion
- Reduces or eliminates asthma symptoms
- Reduces or eliminates cold and flu illnesses
- Cures acne
- Treats yeast infections
- Promotes a natural feeling of well-being
- Acts as a strong, natural antibiotic—without side effects
- Replenishes the body with good bacteria after antibiotic use
- Treats diarrhea
- Helps lactose intolerance
- Promotes deep sleep
- Helps balance blood sugar
- Lowers blood pressure
- Supports the immune system
- Eliminates acid reflux

Even though it's been around for thousands of years, kombucha has recently made an impressive comeback. In fact, estimates are that the kombucha industry will pull in about $500 million in 2015. It has exploded on the market and is causing quite a sensation around the world. You can find this delicious beverage almost anywhere—there are even some fun kombucha bars with imaginative flavor combinations popping up around the country.

Kombucha contains acetic acid, which helps stabilize blood sugar. It also contains an analgesic (pain reliever) and antiarthritic compounds that help remove toxins that may have accumulated in joints, causing pain and inflammation. Kombucha also assists the liver in removing toxins. How does it do this? By binding with toxins and ushering them out of the body. This mechanism was shown in a two-year study on kombucha done by Michael R. Roussin, which involved chemical analysis of 1,103 kombucha samples from all over North America and even some from Europe. He found that glucuronic acid, a powerful detoxifier once thought to be in kombucha, is not present, but derivatives called glucuronides are, and these are what account for the detoxifying power of kombucha.[1]

You might notice, as I did, that in addition to helping detoxify your body, kombucha can help you lose a lot of excess water weight. I have seen it help people eliminate the excess swelling and fluid that accumulates in their tissues from chemical-laden foods and alcohol that can be toxic to the body.

Just like kefir, kombucha has lots of impressive bacteria, but it also has special probiotic yeasts that cannot be killed by antibiotics.

The powerful yeast *Saccharomyces boulardii*, which is abundant in kombucha, was discovered by French microbiologist Henri Boulard in the late 1920s. He was looking for a yeast that would withstand heat for making wine when he happened upon it. In his research of the yeast, he found that it had multiple protective effects for rats infected with cholera. And when Boulard himself became a victim of cholera, he found that he could stop the associated diarrhea by drinking a tea that contained this yeast.

His discovery improved gastrointestinal (GI) health across the board, and *S. boulardii* became the most thoroughly researched of all of probiotic supplements.[2] It is now used to treat *Clostridium difficile*, acute diarrhea, antibiotic-associated diarrhea, some parasitic forms of diarrhea, and other gastrointestinal disorders.[3] It also has a record of helping reduce the symptoms of irritable bowel syndrome (IBS). I got to see the healing power of kombucha firsthand when my daughter Maci alleviated her IBS and healed her leaky gut, in part, by drinking a glass of kombucha with lunch and dinner every day.

This special yeast also has anti-inflammatory and antitoxin effects. It neutralizes toxins produced by harmful pathogens and sends out a signal to the body to reduce inflammation, which can lead to a number of negative health outcomes. Interestingly enough, *S. boulardii* can also act as a decoy to harmful pathogens. It attracts and binds with the pathogens, keeping them from attaching to the intestinal wall and doing damage.

One of the most interesting things about *S. boulardii* is that it is resistant to stomach acid and cannot be killed by antibiotics, which makes it incredibly useful for maintaining a healthy gut when treating an illness with antibiotics. Antibiotics do not target only bad bacteria; they target all bacteria, so your internal ecosystem can easily get thrown off. Many people suggest taking a probiotic supplement to replenish the good bacteria, but stomach acid kills many of these. (Cultured foods are different. Their good bacteria survive stomach acid because the food provides a protective halo.) This can leave us in a vulnerable state. So *S. boulardii* comes to the rescue. It can survive and help keep the gut in balance. But keep in mind that *S. boulardii* doesn't stay in the body indefinitely. It lasts only about two or three days, so you will need to replenish it regularly. This shouldn't be a problem once you taste how delicious kombucha is.

Many have heard that kombucha is not good for people who have an abundance of the harmful yeast candida. But I have found the opposite to be true—as long as the kombucha is made properly. Kombucha can cause problems if it is not fermented long enough and not all the sugar has been removed. Sugar is actually the problem for those with candida because sugar feeds candida. If kombucha is made correctly, the bacteria and yeasts consume the sugars, and as they ferment the by-products are probiotics. How cool is that? You get less sugar, and they make probiotics for you.

CULTURED VEGETABLES

Of all the cultured foods I make, cultured veggies are the most beautiful. They sit on my counter fermenting, and everybody who sees them exclaims, "What are those?!" The vibrant colors and textures are just one benefit—they also taste delicious and give you loads of energy, plus they're jam-packed with healthy bacteria.

Making cultured vegetables is as easy as submerging vegetables in water. When you do this, the veggies make their own lactic acid bacteria, which changes their environment, increasing vitamin C and flooding the vegetables with good bacteria that can even remove pesticides and harmful chemicals in the vegetables themselves.[4] And if you use a culture packet to kick-start fermentation, you can get an even more powerful product.

Cultured vegetables are so potent that all you need is one small spoonful to get billions of probiotics. These

NOTED HEALTH BENEFITS OF KOMBUCHA

- Assists the liver in cleansing and detoxifying
- Helps with weight loss
- Supports the immune system
- Boosts energy
- Prevents kidney stones
- Prevents cancer
- Protects the lining of the stomach
- Has antibiotic-resistant probiotic yeast

microbes then work like an army, killing pathogens and keeping your gut in balance. One of the most powerful guys in there is *Lactobacillus plantarum.* This bacterium is able to overpower many bad bacteria by taking the nutrients they need to survive. This weakens the harmful bacteria and prevents them from attaching to the mucosal lining of your intestines.

If you read my first book, *Cultured Food for Life,* you know how cultured vegetables became a staple in my life. My husband, my oldest daughter, and I were all pretty sick from food poisoning (and not, may I note, from eating a cultured food). I became so sick that I felt delusional. I couldn't think straight and was having a hard time breathing. The room was spinning and I was scared. I remember lying in bed, going in and out of sleep, and dreaming about chickens, of all things. As I woke up from my dream I remembered something I had read earlier that week. It was a story of some chickens that were cured of bird flu with a diet of fermented vegetables.[5] I had made my first jar of cultured veggies that same week. They were just sitting in the back of the fridge. Could I get to the kitchen to eat some? I remember hanging on to the walls as I made my way there. I was so dizzy, and the toxins were making me unable to stay upright for long, but I managed to find the jar and open it. I was too weak to get a spoon from the other side of the kitchen, so I just swigged some juice from the jar and made my way back to bed.

Twenty minutes later I was up doing dishes in the kitchen and feeling almost normal. I remember thinking that I had just experienced a miracle, and I found myself crying over the sink.

I have seen the healing power of cultured vegetables many times now. Friends and family have all experienced the ability of these foods to knock out stomach viruses, colds, and flu. Everyone knows what it's like to have stomach cramps and diarrhea. It's miserable, and I know of nothing (including medication) that is more effective at curing this than cultured veggies. Simply take one spoonful of juice every hour and it will stop your illness in its tracks, speeding you on your way to wellness. You just have to turn to your fridge for help.

Now that you know about my three good friends, let's take a quick look at some of their good friends: prebiotics.

NOTED HEALTH BENEFITS OF CULTURED VEGETABLES

- Stop diarrhea and constipation
- Support adrenals
- Help with weight loss
- Reduce candida
- Reduce or eliminates allergies
- Help ease the symptoms of bowel disease
- Reduce inflammation
- Combat colds and flu
- Alleviate the symptoms of food poisoning

CHAPTER 3

Prebiotics: Another Digestive Ally

Health is never mere chance.
It's the result of forces working together.

Do you remember when eating fiber became the new craze and fiber was put in everything? I never understood this, since the body can't absorb fiber. Yes, it keeps things moving along through the colon to speed elimination, but how does it help the body's immune system—one of the big claims being made?

The answer is prebiotics, which in the last few years have become nearly as popular as probiotics. But what are prebiotics? In short, they are food for the healthy bacteria in our gut. This food makes the bacteria stronger and better able to multiply. Prebiotics come in the form of indigestible fiber in many of the fruits and vegetables we consume. While our bodies cannot digest the fiber in these prebiotic foods, our bacteria can—and we receive the benefits. Having strong, healthy bacteria leads to a balanced gut, which is essential for a good immune system. That's how fiber helps! Prebiotics have also been shown to increase our ability to absorb calcium, magnesium, and other minerals usually lacking in our diets.

Prebiotics are found mostly in fruits and vegetables, including bananas, berries, kale, chard, onions, garlic, leeks, asparagus, artichokes, jicama, chicory root, dandelion greens; some whole grains; honey; and some say even milk. Prebiotics can also be put into food products and supplements with names such as inulin and fructo-oligosaccharides.

Probiotics can be killed by heat, which means that if you cook the foods containing them, you kill the bacteria and lose the beneficial effects. However, prebiotics aren't as fragile, so you can lightly cook them and still get the benefits. This opens up a whole host of eating possibilities. Personally, I love to add a few of my favorite prebiotic supplements and sweeteners—Prebio Plus and SweetLeaf Stevia (powder form)—to my hot foods and drinks. It not only nourishes the good bacteria in my gut but also adds a touch of sweetness that I really enjoy.

I have also been adding prebiotics to my cultured vegetables when I'm in the process of making them—and I've had wonderful results. When you make cultured vegetables with a culture, I often recommend adding a small amount of some kind of prebiotic sweetener to awaken the bacteria in the cultures, making them more abundant. And recently I have found that if my kefir overferments, separating and becoming too sour, I can use the prebiotic Prebio Plus to fix it. Just add, shake, and then place your kefir in the fridge; it will be creamy and delicious the next morning.

The power of prebiotics is currently being shown in a large study on pre- and probiotics called the American Gut Project. It's the world's largest open-source science project aiming to understand the microbial diversity of the human gut. In the project, people send in samples of their bacteria in different forms. The project provides them with a list of the bacteria in their samples—and shows them how their bacterial community compares with others.

As part of this project, the researchers traveled to Tanzania, where they began studying the Hadza, a hunter-forager group whose members still hunt the same animals and gather the same plants that our ancestors did for millions of years. Since they don't eat the processed, sugar-laden foods of the modern diet, the researchers thought the Hadza might hold in their guts some important clues to what an optimal gut microbiome might look like.

One thing they found is that the Hadza people have many different types of bacteria from the foods they eat and the way they prepare them, and from the environment the live in. This diversity is likely the reason they are free of most Western diseases. Researchers also found that even though their diet changes a great deal according to the

GOOD PREBIOTIC SOURCES

- Apples
- Artichokes
- Asparagus
- Bananas
- Barley
- Beans
- Berries
- Bran
- Broccoli
- Brussels sprouts
- Burdock root
- Cabbage
- Carrots
- Cauliflower
- Chard
- Chicory root
- Collard greens
- Dandelion greens
- Garlic
- Honey
- Jicama
- Kale
- Leeks
- Legumes
- Onions
- Radishes
- Rutabaga
- Rye
- Squash
- Sweet potatoes
- Whole wheat

season—they have a wet and a dry season—the bacteria in their guts stay strong, diverse, and happy. It seems that this is due to the consistent intake of fibrous tubers—prebiotics—in the Hadza diet. They don't have to constantly replenish the different types of bacteria to keep the diversity; they simply maintain it through prebiotics.

The researcher Jeff Leach, who lived among the Hadza, wanted to see the effect that this diet would have on him, so he tested himself and found that he could change his gut bacteria in a day with the amount of soluble fiber he consumed.[1] This was very exciting to me, so I started experimenting on myself by eating a lot of prebiotics. When I did this, an interesting thing happened: I started to crave certain fruits and vegetables as never before. One craving would last for a few days or weeks, and then a different one would appear. First it was avocados, then kiwifruit, and then celery and broccoli (dipped in kefir cheese, of course). Weeks later it was leeks and artichokes. What I found was that the more prebiotics I ate, the more I wanted them. It was like a good health spiral. How cool is that?

Interestingly, the power of prebiotics has always been influencing my life, but I didn't know it. When I was introducing you to kombucha, I told you about my daughter Maci and how she repaired her damaged gut, but I didn't give you the whole story. I mentioned that she drank kombucha daily, but what I didn't say is that this was part of a strict daily regimen of consuming all parts of the Trilogy (more on that later). She was also doing something else that was equally important—though we didn't know it at the time: she was eating a lot of prebiotics. Maci loved coffee but it hurt her stomach. I had found a delicious tea that worked as a substitute, but I didn't know it was loaded with prebiotics. It had dandelion root and chicory root (which is inulin), and she drank it every day. I was also making her leek soup, and leeks are huge prebiotics. These items, along with the cultured foods, allowed her good bacteria to grow like crazy, and her pain went away. I wish I had known then what I know now.

Eating prebiotics along with cultured foods is the one-two punch that allows your good bacteria to be all they can be.

CHAPTER 4

Your Health and Cultured Foods

"The greatest medicine of all is to teach people how not to need it."
—Anonymous

This was the hardest part of the book for me to write. It's a chapter that lists all sorts of diseases—along with the science showing how the bacteria in cultured foods can help prevent them. I guess ultimately it's not about disease, but it felt that way when I was writing it.

I believe so strongly in wellness that I don't like to focus on disease. It's not an easy thing for me because so often people discuss illness as if it's the norm, all the while forgetting that wellness should be the most prominent state of being. This outlook disempowers people and makes them feel as if they don't know what's right for them. Years ago, I was often influenced by well-meaning friends and family and the media. They scared me to death with the latest news they had heard, saying things like "Don't eat that!" and "Did you read that story about how bad this food is for you?" It drove me crazy trying to figure out what to believe. Finally I'd had enough. They didn't know any better than I did, so I decided to follow my own path, seek my own guidance from within, and forget what everybody else thought was right for me.

So why am I writing about diseases—writing an entire, *long* chapter about illness? It's because I think it's important for you to hear about the incredible science that links good health and the bacteria you find in cultured foods. Think of this chapter as being not about disease but about inspiration. I am bound and determined to make my books and my business about all the wonderful things you should do, not the scary things you shouldn't do. By showing you just how powerful bacteria are, I hope to convince you that cultured foods can be your best friends. This is by no means an exhaustive list of illnesses, nor is it an account of all the science that's out there, but it will open your eyes to some of the things happening in the scientific community. More and more research surfaces every day, and it's so exciting to see that science is recognizing the power of the gut.

Just remember, when you have an ailment of any kind, the illness is not the enemy; it's a sign from your body that it needs your help to correct something. If you're like most people, you will go to the doctor and, most of the time, take medication to mask a symptom rather than correct the underlying problem. Please pay attention to your body's cries for help. And if you have any of these ailments, please don't be discouraged but rather turn to your heart, mind, and body to find the solution.

So let's jump right into this list of your body's communications!

Acid Reflux/Gastroesophageal Reflux Disease (GERD)

A man named John came up to me after one of my classes and said, "I take a glass of kefir every day before I go to work—without fail. I don't sweeten it. I just drink it straight. I wanted to thank you because it allowed me to get off all my medication for acid reflux. I feel like a new man after years of struggle with this." Then he smiled, shook my hand, and said, "Kefir is powerful medicine for acid reflux, and you should tell everybody who will listen." I am heeding those words because I have heard time and time again how much kefir helps people who are struggling with acid reflux.

Gastroesophageal reflux disease (GERD) occurs when the lower esophageal sphincter malfunctions, allowing the contents of the stomach to flow up into the esophagus. Some speculate that overgrowth of bad bacteria in the stomach causes undigested food to ferment. In turn, this fermentation causes gas to build up, eventually forcing the contents of the stomach up into the esophagus. This is what creates the symptoms of burning and pain commonly associated with acid reflux.

If you are experiencing these symptoms, one of the first things you should do is add fermented foods to your diet to restore balance in your gut. Kefir has been very effective in helping many people with acid reflux. It is packed with the *Lactobacillus* bacterium, which changes your gut flora and reduces the symptoms of acid reflux.

One 2014 study looking at the effect of probiotics on GERD involved 589 infants who were randomly given the probiotic *Lactobacillus reuteri* or a placebo for 90 days. The researchers asked that parents make a daily record of three things: the number of episodes of regurgitation, the number of minutes of inconsolable crying, and the number of bowel movements. The infants who received the probiotics had less crying time, fewer episodes of regurgitation, and significantly less constipation than the control group.[1]

Another insight about reflux deals with the pathogenic bacterium *H. pylori*, which you'll read more about in the ulcer section of this chapter. Until recently, *H. pylori* has been put forth as a "bad" bacterium, but now an interesting twist in its story has been discovered: *H. pylori* protects against acid reflux. As I have said throughout this book, we are seeking balance, so it doesn't surprise me that *H. pylori* can be helpful if it is kept in check.

Martin J. Blaser, M.D., elaborates on the research around *H. pylori* in his book *Missing Microbes*. He says that, when present in large numbers, this bacterium can cause ulcers and even stomach cancer in some people. But *H. pylori* also helps regulate stomach acidity, which plays a large part in the symptoms of GERD. When an ulcer occurs, the standard treatment is using antibiotics to eradicate *H. pylori*, which heals the ulcers but also raises the acidity of the stomach. Blaser and his colleagues found that the patients without *H. pylori* were eight times more likely to have acid reflux.[2] So the treatment that eliminated *H. pylori* worsened acid reflux and even esophageal cancer.

So what to do? Balance your gut with prebiotic and probiotic foods. Keep *H. pylori* in check by adding lots of beneficial microbes that allow *all* your bacteria to work for you. If you have lots of good microbes, the ones that might get out of hand will stay in balance. I would also recommend cutting out refined foods and sugars from your diet, as these change the bacteria species in your gut, causing cravings and addictions for unhealthy foods.[3] It's not as hard as it seems, and you will find that a lot of problems will simply vanish when you change what you eat. Cultured foods plus whole, real, natural sources of nutrition will allow your body to do what it was designed to do: heal itself.

Cultured foods have eliminated acid reflux in many people I have met, including my husband, and the studies that continue to surface give me great hope that soon cultured foods and probiotics will be seen as a viable treatment for this ailment.

Acne

When my youngest daughter, Holli, hit puberty and was flooded with hormones, I learned a lot about acne. Whenever she ate sugar, she would get painful, embarrassing pimples. Knowing that bacteria can cause pimples to flare up, I put her on an all-out, intense cultured food diet to clear out any bad bacteria from her gut. Holli's acne got worse when I flooded her with cultured foods, and after about a week of having the Trilogy in her diet every day, Holli got what at first I thought was a virus. For a few hours she threw up and had diarrhea, and then suddenly it stopped. Holli's skin cleared up the next day, after months of struggle. I believe that Holli was having a healing crisis (more on that in the next chapter), and what I thought was a virus was actually her body's way of getting rid of the pathogens in her gut. This took the pressure off of her largest detoxifier—her skin.

Chris Kresser, M.S., L.Ac., a recognized leader in the fields of functional and integrative medicine, has written, "I'm still waiting to find a patient with skin issues who has no gut issues and no history of gut issues. I haven't seen that yet. I'm not saying they don't exist, but so far everybody I've treated with a skin issue has a gut issue."[4]

One study that draws this connection comes from more than 70 years ago, when dermatologists John H. Stokes and Donald M. Pillsbury proposed a connection between gastrointestinal health and skin conditions such as acne. In their study, Stokes and Pillsbury suggested that emotional states might alter the normal gut flora and increase intestinal permeability, which can contribute to systemic inflammation. Among the remedies advocated by Stokes and Pillsbury was *Lactobacillus acidophilus* cultures.[5]

A much more recent study showed the skin-gut connection as well. This research, which involved more than 13,000 adolescents, found that those with acne were more likely to experience gastrointestinal symptoms such as constipation, halitosis, and gastric reflux.[6]

And do you remember that yeast in kombucha, *S. boulardii*? That has been found to have many benefits for the skin. In a randomized, controlled, double-blind study involving 139 patients with acne, subjects were given this probiotic yeast for five months. More than 80 percent of those in the *S. boulardii* group were considerably or completely improved, while in the placebo group only 26 percent of subjects were improved.

Without question, what goes on in the gut has a huge connection to the skin. When you begin to fix your gut, your skin problems will likely begin to vanish.

Allergies (Seasonal)

When you have a reaction to a harmless substance like pollen, it is because your body sees this substance as a foreign invader and overreacts by sending out inflammatory substances to fight it. This inflammation is what causes your allergy symptoms. The over-reaction means that something is amiss, and we need to figure out what that is. For me, seasonal allergies were a huge sign that something was wrong. I was allergic to pollen for more than 30 years, and finding the way to heal myself was monumental.

The connection between healthy gut flora and allergies was directly shown in a study by immunologist Gary Huffnagle and his colleagues at the University of Michigan. In this experiment, a group of mice were given antibiotics in an effort to disturb the natural bacteria levels in their systems. After the bacteria were killed off, the scientists threw off the balance of the microbiome even more by feeding the mice the yeast *Candida albicans*. The resulting low bacteria-high yeast ratio approximates the conditions of having a yeast infection, which is a sure sign of a gut imbalance. This group of mice and a control group were then exposed to spores of the mold *Aspergillus fumigatus* and to egg white protein—two substances known to cause allergic reactions. The mice in the control group, whose gut bacteria were undisturbed, had a much milder reaction to the allergens than those that had been treated with antibiotics.[7]

Another study was done on people with seasonal allergic rhinitis (SAR). Ten people in a double-blind study were given a milk drink with the probiotic *Lactobacillus casei Shirota* over a period of five months. Ten others were given a placebo. Blood samples were collected before, during, and after peak grass pollen season in order to see how the drink affected those who were treated with the probiotic. The tests showed a significant reduction in levels of antigen immune responses in the treated group, compared with those taking the placebo. In essence, the probiotic supplement reduced the immune system's response to the allergens.[8]

One additional way that cultured foods help reduce the symptoms of allergies is by strengthening the function of the adrenal glands, which produce a variety of hormones including cortisol. Cortisol helps mitigate the inflammation that causes allergy symptoms, and stressed or unhealthy adrenals will produce less cortisol.[9] To remain healthy, adrenal glands need huge amounts of C and B vitamins. Cultured foods, especially kefir and cultured veggies, have lots of vitamin C. (In fact, Captain James Cook, the famous British ship commander, conquered the scourge of scurvy—which is caused by a vitamin C deficiency—by giving his crew fermented sauerkraut on long voyages.)

Consuming vitamins is important, but this isn't the only way cultured vegetables provide good adrenal support. Healthy gut flora is the number-one thing your body needs in order to absorb and use B vitamins, which in turn strengthen your adrenal glands. In fact, healthy gut flora will actually synthesize B vitamins, enzymes, and proteins. When the gut flora are out of balance, this production is impaired.

I personally experience the power of cultured vegetables during allergy season every year. If I'm feeling sick, I simply drink some of the juice, and it makes me feel better in 20 minutes—even when pollen and allergy season is in full swing. I'm like a new woman!

Asthma

One of the very first people I told about cultured foods was my friend Paula. Her little boy had terrible asthma, and we discovered that when he drank kefir every day his asthma went away and he didn't need his inhaler. It had such an impact on this seven-year-old that he would stand in the kitchen and cry that he needed his kefir when he had gone for a few days without it. He knew it was keeping his asthma under control, as he could feel symptoms return when he went without it.

I heard about similar success when I ran into a lady at the grocery store who had come to one of my classes. She told me that her husband had gotten off his inhaler after 15 years of using it, just by adding kefir and cultured veggies to his diet.

Interested in why this was happening, I started to research and found that cases of asthma have increased like crazy in the past 30 years. And then I found a very telling study published in the *American Journal of Epidemiology* that tied asthma to antibiotics. This study found that when doctors give young children antibiotics, their risk of developing asthma before the age of six increases by 50 percent![10] In another study, researchers in the U.K., led by allergist Adnan Custovic, analyzed data from more than 1,000 children from birth until the age of 11. They looked at their medical records to determine how often doctors gave them antibiotics and how often they ended up with asthma. "We noted significantly higher risk of physician-confirmed wheezing after antibiotic prescription," they wrote. There was a 70 percent increase of risk for any kind of asthma case after the use of anti-biotics.[11] This speaks to the connection between healthy gut bacteria and the occurrence of asthma.

Cultured foods help restore the good bacteria that antibiotics destroy. They also re-duce inflammation throughout the body, thus helping open up the constricted airway that is a hallmark of asthma.

Autism

When I was at the beginning of my journey exploring cultured foods, I met Mary. Mary had several boys with severe autism, and she had taken these boys from barely speaking and functioning to thriving. These boys and my kids had drama classes together, so luckily I got the chance to be around Mary each week. She and I would talk for hours on end about cultured foods and microbes, and she would tell me how kefir and cultured vegetables—along with physical therapy—greatly contributed to healing her boys' au-tism. Mary was smart as a whip and understood the science about bacteria. She actually made science seem fun. I will always be grateful to Mary for being a kindred spirit who advanced my desire to learn. Her stories convinced me early on that I needed to learn as much as I could about these cultured foods and help others do the same. So let's look at some of the science of cultured foods and autism.

Everyone is looking for the reason for the dramatic increase in autism in recent years. Many theories have been proposed, from vaccines to viruses, but one of the more convincing is the "hygiene hypothesis," which basically says that we have become too clean. We kill bacteria left and right with rounds and rounds of antibiotics and cleaning supplies, and kids are indoors 24/7. They aren't being exposed to the many kinds of bacteria that lead to a balanced and healthy gut. Interestingly, 90 percent of children with autism have some kind of gastrointestinal symptom or digestive problem.

One study on autism that really made an impact on me was done by food microbiologist Glenn Gibson at the University of Reading. It is referred to by some people as "the trial that was so successful, it failed." The study was done with 40 autistic children all between the ages of 4 and 13 years. Each child was randomly placed in one of two groups. For three weeks one group was given a probiotic supplement with the species *Lactobacillus plantarum*, which is abundant in cultured vegetables. The other children were given a placebo. After three weeks the researchers planned to switch what each group was receiving, supplement or placebo. However, the parents of the children taking the probiotic saw such positive results that they knew which group they were in and refused to switch to the placebo. They saw too many improvements in not only digestive health but also mental and behavioral health that they said it was heartbreaking to have to stop their child from taking the probiotic. The children were calmer and had a greater ability to listen and concentrate. The trial had such a large dropout rate that it was discontinued.[12]

In another study, which was done on mice at the California Institute of Technology, researchers found that mothers who had an induced infection or inflammation during pregnancy had offspring with autism-like behaviors, such as social avoidance, anxiety, repetitive actions, and GI disorders. The researchers fed these mice *Bacteroides fragilis*, a bacterium that has been used as in probiotic therapy in animals with GI disorders and is also found in a healthy human gut. The result? The behavior of the treated mice changed. They were more likely to interact with other mice, had reduced anxiety, and were less likely to become aggressive.[13]

I can't tell you how important I think cultured foods are for autism and many other childhood diseases. We aren't talking about drugs; we are talking about food—cultured foods. You have to feed your children something, so why not try to add cultured foods to their diets? It could make all the difference, and just like the parents in the University of Reading study, you would need no further evidence. Changing what you eat works!

Cancer/Chemotherapy

There are many studies that show cultured foods help in the prevention and treatment of cancer. The multiple strains of good bacteria and yeasts in kefir, kombucha, and cultured vegetables have the ability to detoxify the foods you ingest that have carcinogens.

They also help boost the immune system and create an environment hostile to carcinogenic poisons that can cause cancer.

In 2005 a team of researchers in Poland and the United States studied two groups of young Polish women: one that had immigrated to the United States and one that had not. They found that the rate of breast cancer was three times higher for those in the United States than for those still living in Poland. Further studies concluded that the consumption of cultured sauerkraut was a possible factor in the differing rates of cancer. The women in Poland ate an average of 30 pounds of cultured sauerkraut each year, while the women in the United States ate less than 10 pounds per year.[14] Why does this matter? Sauerkraut contains high levels of glucosinolates, which have been shown to have anticancer activity in laboratory research.

Other studies have focused on estrogen metabolism and the enzymes in sauerkraut and its juices. A 2012 study conducted by biochemist Hanna Szaefer and her colleagues looked at the ability of the enzymes in cabbage and sauerkraut to change the expression of the P450 enzyme, which metabolizes estrogen but is also carcinogenic. Their research supported the idea that the consumption of sauerkraut was beneficial for the prevention of breast cancer in women.[15]

There have been a few recent studies that have directly linked the consumption of kefir to improvement in cancer cases. In 2011 one study showed that kefir reduced the damage to the DNA in colorectal cancers and colon cancer.[16] Another study showed that cancer cells in the stomach started to mutate and self-destruct with the addition of kefir to the diet.[17] And in another, researchers gave kefir to mice daily and found that it was very effective in regulating the immune system and stopping breast cancer growth.[18]

Along with cancer often comes the use of chemotherapy, which brings with it a host of other problems. There has been some research done on the connection between the gut and chemo. In one clinical study, researchers gave a group of mice an injection of chemotherapy that would, pound for pound, kill most adult human beings. Why? As Jian-Guo Geng, associate professor at the University of Michigan School of Dentistry, said, "All tumors from different tissues and organs can be killed by high doses of chemotherapy and radiation, but the current challenge for treating the later-staged metastasized cancer is that you actually kill the [patient] before you kill the tumor." So the goal was to test a recently discovered biological mechanism that focuses on preserving the integrity of the gastrointestinal tract—a mechanism that helped mice live through this lethal dose of chemotherapy.

The mice were injected with a substance called Rspo1, or R-spondon1, which activates stem cell production within the gut. These stem cells then rebuild damaged tissue faster than chemo can destroy it. Of the mice that were given R-spondon1, 50 to 75 percent survived the potentially fatal chemotherapy dose. All the mice in the control group died.[19] Here is the exciting part: Your body already has a way to make R-spondon1 on its own. Inside the human gut, a layer of epithelial cells is regenerated every four to five days, as long as you have the right gut flora. If your gut flora are healthy and include a group of healthy strains of bacteria, your body will regenerate itself. If they do not, then it slows or halts the regeneration of your intestinal cells. The probiotics in your gut can determine how and if your body survives chemotherapy—making it even more crucial for those with cancer and going through chemo to add cultured foods and prebiotics to their diets.

Cancer and chemotherapy are complex and affect people in different ways. I am certainly not saying that cultured foods are a cure-all, but rather encouraging you to change what you eat and include probiotic and whole, real foods. You're the captain of your ship; steer wisely.

Colds and Flu

Throughout the past 13 years I have watched my body get stronger and stronger as my immune system has been strengthened by the foods I eat and the lifestyle choices I make. When I am around people with colds and flus, I am no longer afraid I will get a cold or the flu, too. I actually like the fact that my body is exposed to these types of germs because it makes my immune system stronger.

So why am I not afraid of getting a cold or the flu? It's the strength of our immune system that determines whether you get sick, and cultured foods help boost the immune system.

Researchers at Harvard Medical School have found evidence of a relationship between good bacteria and the immune system. Certain bacteria in the gut influence the development of the immune system by doing such things as correcting deficiencies and increasing the number of something called T cells. There are two kinds of T cells: killers and helpers. Killer T cells find and destroy infected cells that have been turned into virus-making factories. Helper T cells don't fight invaders themselves. Instead, they are like team coordinators. When a helper T cell sends out a chemical message, its matched killer T cell is alerted that there is a virus present and seeks to destroy it. Having lots of good bacteria in the gut increases T cell production and keeps communication among all the cells functioning.[20]

In an article in *Penn Medicine*, David Artis, Ph.D., associate professor of microbiology at the Perelman School of Medicine at the University of Pennsylvania, notes that bacteria are essential to fight off viral infections. "From our studies in mice, we found that signals derived from these beneficial microbes are essential for optimal immune responses to experimental viral infections," says Artis. "In one way we could consider these microbes as our 'brothers in arms' in the fight against infectious diseases."

To come to this conclusion, Artis's lab treated mice with antibiotics to reduce the number of bacteria in their guts. These mice were then subjected to the influenza virus, and the outcome was telling. The mice had an impaired immune response to the virus, and the virus didn't leave their bodies as quickly as it left those in the control group. The mice also had severely damaged airways and an increased rate of death.[21]

So as you can see, these invisible microbes really are our brothers in arms, fighting unseen battles as we go through our days.

Colitis

I receive lots of e-mails and Facebook posts from people who have been greatly helped or healed from colitis by consuming cultured foods. Ulcerative colitis is inflammation of the colon and rectum that causes tiny open sores to form. This can lead to diarrhea, bloody stools, abdominal pain, and cramping.

Probiotics are used often to treat colitis, and now there is a surge in fecal transplants, which have been approved by the FDA to restore good bacteria to the colon. The concept is to give one person's healthy bacteria to another by transferring healthy feces through the rectum and colon. Sounds intense, right? But here's the deal: there's a much less frightening way to accomplish this. You eat probiotic and prebiotic foods and change the microbiome inside of you. Probiotics naturally act as a barrier to the intestinal lining, keeping inflammation down. They increase mucus production to create a thicker mucus layer, which protects against invasive bacteria.

In one study, 34 patients with mild to moderate ulcerative colitis who had not responded to conventional therapy underwent six weeks of treatment with the high-potency probiotic mixture VSL#3, which contains eight strains of probiotics, many of which are found in cultured foods: *Bifidobacterium breve, Bifidobacterium longum, Bifidobacterium infantis, Lactobacillus acidophilus, Lactobacillus plantarum, Lactobacillus paracasei, Lactobacillus bulgaricus,* and *Streptococcus thermophilus.*

The outcome was impressive: 77 percent of participants responded to the probiotic treatment. And there were none of the adverse effects that often accompany conventional treatment.[22]

Another study—a double-blind study of 144 patients who had mild to moderate ulcerative colitis and were already being treated with 5-aminosalicylic acid (5-ASA) and/or immunosuppressants—split participants into two sets. For eight weeks, one group used the same VSL#3 mixture noted in the study above and the other took a placebo. The probiotic group saw a greater reduction in their scores on the ulcerative colitis disease activity index (UCDAI), a scale used to measure symptom activity in ulcerative colitis, than the placebo group. In other words, the people on the probiotics had better results from their treatments compared with those who were being treated only with ASA or immunosuppressants. Researchers also found the probiotics improved rectal bleeding, and if the patient relapsed, reintroducing the probiotics again for eight weeks caused the patients to go back into remission.[23]

These studies are very exciting, but there's nothing quite as inspiring to me as the firsthand accounts I hear. This is a testimony from someone who actually healed from colitis by using cultured foods.

> It's strange that my colitis disease is something I have kept hidden from my closest friends, who had no idea what I've been through since 1976 . . . I was soooo excited to be able to tell my specialist that my colitis of 38 years is under control. No blood. No urgency. No mucus. With my latest relapse being my worst ever, I had been going five to six times before work just to empty my bowels so I could keep my new job, which I love.
>
> When I queried the new, stronger immunosuppressant drug [my doctor] wanted me on, I chose to reject it after research. Why would I reduce my autoimmune system to reduce inflammation when my immune system is the one part I want strong?
>
> From the moment I was gifted your book *Cultured Food for Life* and some milk kefir grains, I set out on a journey of discovery of probiotics and good gut flora. My aim was to reduce my dependence on immunosuppressant drugs. Through the ease of following the Trilogy of milk kefir, kombucha, and veggie ferments, I now have a quality of life that I never thought possible.

Crohn's Disease

Jordan Rubin, health advocate and founder of Garden of Life, Inc., wasn't always the thriving entrepreneur he is today. I heard him speak at a conference and found out that his successful company was born from the pain he endured with Crohn's disease. As a 19-year-old, he was diagnosed with Crohn's, which nearly ended his life. Before Crohn's, he was 6'1" and 180 pounds. After suffering with this condition, he got to a low of 104 pounds and was confined to a wheelchair. He crossed the world, visiting dozens of health professionals and trying more than 300 supplements, and he just continued to get worse. So he started studying nutrition and changed his diet to include only whole, living, enzyme- and probiotic-rich foods. He said he drank two quarts of kefir a day and consumed many other fermented foods and supplements. Within four months, he had regained his weight and his body began to heal. It's been many years now, and he exhibits no symptoms of Crohn's. With his health restored he went on to be become a successful author, speaker, certified nutritional consultant, and successful business owner.

So is there any proof that the probiotic additions to Jordan's diet are responsible for his health? Yep. A recent study published in *Genome Medicine* found that people with Crohn's had less diversity in healthy bacteria and more harmful bacteria in their guts. This was linked not only with the subjects' DNA but also with the use of antibiotics. "The intestinal bacteria, or 'gut microbiome,' you develop at a very young age can have a big impact on your health for the rest of your life," lead study author Dan Knights, a University of Minnesota biotechnologist, told *Discover: Science + Technology*. "We have found groups of genes that may play a role in shaping the development of imbalanced gut microbes."[24]

Another study looked at how adding good microbes can help reduce inflammation in people with Crohn's. In this study, *Lactobacillus casei* or *Lactobacillus bulgaricus* were cultured with specimens of tissue taken from ten patients with Crohn's. In the tissue that was inflamed, the bacteria slowed the production of the cytokines responsible for the inflammation.[25]

Depression

There is a lot of research linking an unhealthy gut to depression. The gut, sometimes called the "second brain," contains a hundred million neurons, more than in either the spinal cord or the peripheral nervous system. A combination of nerves, hormones, bacteria, blood, and the organs of the digestive system handle the complex task of breaking down our food, absorbing nutrients, and expelling wastes—all the while keeping our immune system strong. Since digestion requires a considerable amount of the body's energy, when it starts to struggle we can feel it in our emotions.

Michael Gershon, chairman of the Department of Anatomy and Cell Biology at New York–Presbyterian Hospital/Columbia University Medical Center and an expert in neuro-gastroenterology, says, "Everyday emotional well-being may rely on messages from the brain below to the brain above."[26] The reason the gut and mood are so intimately intertwined is that the bacteria of the gut produce hundreds of hormones that help regulate the body. While many people think that serotonin—the hormone that produces happy feelings—comes from the brain, the reality is that 95 percent of it is manufactured in the gut.[27] But if your gut isn't balanced, it can't produce this hormone as efficiently. So the kind of microflora you have will in great part determine what kind of moods you have.

But this is great because you can alter the makeup of your microbiome by adding cultured foods. One three-part, placebo-controlled human study showed that adding probiotics can, in fact, decrease anxiety, diminish perceptions of stress, and improve overall mental outlook.[28]

Experimental studies have also shown that supplementing with probiotic bacteria can increase peripheral tryptophan levels. Tryptophan is a precursor to serotonin and dopamine (the other happy hormone), so increased tryptophan means increased serotonin and dopamine.[29]

More and more studies are surfacing each day that show that as our diets have changed to include more chemical preservatives, the number of depression cases has also risen. We no longer eat the foods that help keep our guts in balance, so it's no surprise that our bodies have rebelled. I found myself experiencing depression without even realizing what was happening. Slowly over time I lost my joy for life, and as I went through my day-to-day routine I started to think that this was normal. But I was wrong! We are supposed to be happy; it's how our bodies are designed. We have all the machinery inside of us to create a feeling of well-being, optimism, and happiness, but it doesn't work correctly if we feed our bodies garbage.

Diabetes

Diabetes is something I saw firsthand in my family as I grew up. Watching this disease (both type 1 and type 2) affect my family left a profound impression on me. So when I developed type 2 diabetes during my last pregnancy—only to watch it disappear and then return again after my daughter's birth—I knew I was in a lot of trouble. I remember how awful I felt. I was exhausted, and my days revolved around finding time to sit on the couch. I knew that if I didn't fix this problem, it would likely take me away from my family much too early. And while it was awful, I am so thankful for the pain that it caused because it made me start seeking answers and take charge of my health. It's also one of the things that led me to cultured foods.

Day-to-day life with diabetes is pretty terrible. It feels like having unseen forces controlling you. You have food cravings and you want to eat large amounts of food. You become accustomed to feeling bad. And in the long term, it can lead to strokes and heart attacks.

I will never forget the day when I felt my diabetes start to reverse. I had been drinking kefir for about a month and I was feeling better, but on that particular day my blood sugars had normalized, and not only did the blood machine say so but so did my body. I was standing in the kitchen, doing dishes, and suddenly found myself in the front yard filling up my bird feeder. I hadn't cared about the birds and their food for weeks, but suddenly I wanted to take care of them—I wanted to take care of everybody. Feelings of well-being and joy enveloped me like a blanket. I knew my body was healing and letting me know I was on the right path.

So how does eating probiotic foods help with diabetes?

Many studies are confirming that altered gut flora are present in humans and animals with obesity, insulin resistance, diabetes, and hypertension. Growing research suggests that people who are obese and resistant to insulin have microbes in their gut that are different from healthy people's. The leaner you are, the more Firmicutes you have, and the more obese, the more Bacteroidetes.[30]

There is evidence that feeding probiotics and prebiotics to those with diabetes-related obesity and metabolic disorders can dramatically reduce insulin resistance, restore glucose sensitivity, and lower blood pressure and weight by altering their gut flora and encouraging the right kind of microbes to thrive and grow.[31] This simply adds to a feeling of overall well-being. These conditions can be very draining and tax the body, so when you balance your gut, you liberate energy, lifting your mood and outlook on life.

Fibromyalgia

Fibromyalgia is one of the fastest-growing disabling conditions, and it seems to affect mostly women. I see it cropping up everywhere. It is a chronic inflammatory condition that causes muscular and joint pain and extreme fatigue. It is debilitating and can ruin people's lives. More and more evidence is pointing to an unhealthy gut in people suffering from fibromyalgia. One study found that those who have fibromyalgia also have leaky gut syndrome or IBS.[32] Another study showed that 73 percent of patients with fibromyalgia reported gastrointestinal symptoms and signs and that IBS was present in 30 to 70 percent of fibromyalgia patients.[33]

This shows that there is a link between fibromyalgia and gut problems—but not that one is causing the other. However, there is one study that seems to shed light on causation. This study focused on patients with both fibromyalgia and small intestinal bacterial overgrowth (SIBO). Part of the group was treated for SIBO by using antibiotics; the other half got a placebo. In those who were treated, there was a decrease in the symptoms of fibromyalgia—thus suggesting that gut problems cause fibromyalgia.[34] While this one study isn't conclusive, it seems that gut problems could be at the base of fibromyalgia. This, then, suggests that healing the gut would go a long way in helping restore the body back to its natural state.

Anecdotal evidence from people who have come to my classes speaks to the power of cultured foods in helping fibromyalgia. Check out this story from Sherri:

> Over 20 years ago, I was diagnosed with fibromyalgia. For years I've had an all-over body ache that felt like inflammation. It was an ache that I had every day. I was especially achy when we had rainy weather.
>
> After having a terrible bout with a stomach virus that lasted about a week, I searched out information about how to heal my gut issues. I found your videos and that's where it all began.
>
> After watching your videos I immersed myself in making kefir, cultured veggies, and kombucha. After three weeks of filling myself with these wonderful foods, I woke up one morning and realized I didn't have that all-over body ache anymore. It's been that way for the past eight days, and I'm so excited about it. Also, it's calmed my painful gastric problems, and I have a sense of well-being. I know this is something that I'm going to continue to do because it's improving my health.

Food Allergies/Intolerance

I hear about food allergies and food intolerance all the time in my work. Generally, the symptoms of food intolerance (gas, bloating, heartburn, headaches, and so on) are less intense, while the symptoms of food allergies (rashes, hives, shortness of breath, trouble swallowing, chest pain, or a drop in blood pressure) are dramatic.[35] Both food allergies and food intolerance can also cause stomach pain, nausea, vomiting, and diarrhea. In either case, the person who has them lives with great discomfort.

My daughter Maci struggled with food sensitivities for years. When she was 16, she was constantly tired and dealing with the pain and discomfort of general digestive issues. Every week the list of foods that caused stomach distress for her grew longer. We took her to doctor after doctor, each of whom came to the conclusion that she was *probably* dealing with IBS or food allergies, but no one was willing to give a definitive diagnosis. Finally, one doctor suggested that she have surgery to remove her gallbladder, but he couldn't give us a reason why. So I decided to do some research rather than put Maci through a surgery that might not help her. What I discovered was that the lining of Maci's gut was damaged and that years of antibiotics had stripped her of all her good bacteria. This is what was wreaking havoc in her digestive system. This is why she seemed to be allergic to foods.

I devised a plan to heal her gut. We removed all the foods that caused her pain, and she ate a cultured food at every meal, making sure to incorporate all the pieces of the Trilogy. This helped her digest her meals and began to heal her gut. As I mentioned in the last chapter, she was also ingesting all kinds of prebiotics, though we didn't know it at the time. Adding cultured foods and prebiotics gave her many strains of good bacteria and created a new microbiome in her gut. Within a month her stomach stopped hurting. Within three months her so-called food allergies started evaporating, and a year later she could eat anything she desired.

Because of what Maci was going through I started searching everywhere to find evidence of how eating cultured foods healed food allergies, but none was to be found—except the anecdotal evidence I saw with Maci and the many other people I was teaching. *Until now.*

In Chapter 1, I talked a little about an exciting study, published in the *Proceedings of the National Academy of Sciences*, that identified not only a possible cause of food allergies but also a probable cure. The team found that young children overexposed to antibiotics were at greater risk of developing food allergies. They were also able to identify a naturally occurring class of bacteria in the human gut that keeps people from developing those allergies. This class, called *Clostridia*, includes hundreds of members, but it diminishes with frequent antibiotic use at a young age—making children more susceptible to food allergies. Maci received antibiotics every year when she got her annual sinus infection, and now I can see how this affected her.

The research team administered antibiotics to young mice and found they were more likely than the control group to develop peanut allergies. Then they were given *Clostridia*—and like magic, the mice's sensitivity went away. They were no longer allergic.[36]

The increase in allergic diseases seen in industrialized countries is being attributed to the hygiene hypothesis, which I discussed in the autism section—the idea that the overuse of antibiotics, food sterilization, and antibacterial cleaning products has led to a lack of diversity in the microbial strains in infants. Data show that the gut flora in children with allergies are different from those in children without allergies.

High Blood Pressure

Fourteen years ago, before I found cultured foods, my body was sending me clues that something was wrong. I never put it all together until I was in a crisis. I had extremely high blood pressure, and the stress of that—along with my pregnancy—began affecting my liver. My baby was delivered early to save my life, but my blood pressure didn't come down afterward. In the hospital I was on a high-dose magnesium drip that made me so sick I couldn't get out of bed. This meant that I couldn't see my new daughter, who was in the neonatal unit down the hall. It tortured me, and being kept from my daughter made my blood pressure even higher. She was too fragile to leave the neonatal unit, and I couldn't even sit up long enough to get into a wheelchair. It is times like these that can change our lives if we let them. I was begging God to bring my blood pressure down when a nurse came into the room, and I asked her if she would take me to my daughter. I told her it would help lower my blood pressure. So she did just that. At two in the morning, she wheeled my entire bed into the neonatal unit, and there I saw my four-pound preemie.

My blood pressure started to come down following the visit, and as I rested in bed I started putting the pieces together. If I was on a magnesium drip so I wouldn't have a stroke, did that mean my body wasn't hanging on to magnesium? Perhaps this was the cause of my high blood pressure. I started researching this many months later at about the same time I started drinking kefir. With the addition of kefir to my diet, my blood pressure began to normalize. Interestingly, I found out that not only is kefir high in magnesium, but it also helps you absorb more of it from the foods you eat.

Magnesium deficiencies can wreak havoc in more ways than one. Magnesium is a cofactor in more than 800 enzyme systems that regulate different biochemical reactions in the body, including protein synthesis, muscle and nerve function, blood-glucose control, and blood pressure regulation. Magnesium can be found in food, but the amount is dependent upon the concentration in the soil where the food is grown. Highly processed foods, and especially sugar, deplete the body of magnesium. A number of studies have shown that magnesium can benefit your blood pressure and help prevent sudden cardiac arrest, heart attack,[37] and stroke. For example, one meta-analysis, which was published in the *American Journal of Clinical Nutrition*, looked at seven studies that covered more than 240,000 participants. The results showed that dietary magnesium intake is inversely associated with risk of ischemic stroke.[38]

Another study found that kefir works on an enzyme in the stomach to lower blood pressure naturally in one out of three people.[39] It also reduces inflammation throughout the body. And more and more studies are finding that probiotic fermented milk has blood pressure—lowering effects in prehypertensive and hypertensive people.[40]

Adding cultured foods to my diet was a key factor in healing my body from high blood pressure.

High Cholesterol

Many years ago I had several friends tell me that their cholesterol started improving when they began to eat fermented foods. This made them believers in the power and importance of fermented foods. One friend even asked me, "If eating these cultured foods could do this, what would happen if I changed the rest of my diet?" As you've seen so far, the answer is "a lot," including lowering cholesterol.

A double-blind study with 60 volunteers aged 18 to 65 looked at the effects of probiotics on cholesterol. Each day for 12 weeks, one group received a capsule that contained 120 billion viable *Lactobacillus* strains, which happen to be abundant in cultured vegetables. The other group got a placebo. There was a 13.6 percent overall reduction in total cholesterol in the people who took the probiotic, compared with the placebo group. Moreover, the participants with the highest cholesterol at the start of the study reduced their total cholesterol by 17.4 percent. Their LDL cholesterol—the bad cholesterol—was lowered by 17.6 percent, compared with the placebo group.[41] This is a significant reduction in total cholesterol. Ingesting cultured foods provides not only the *Lactobacillus* strains that were used in the study but also various others that add to an overall balanced gut.

Another study gave participants live yogurt with *Lactobacillus*. After six weeks researchers found significant reductions in LDL cholesterol (8.92 percent) and total cholesterol (4.81 percent). The same group performed a second trial with similar results.[42]

One reason probiotics help lower cholesterol is because bacteria consume prebiotic (soluble) fiber in the small intestines and create acids, one of which is called propionic acid. This particular acid reduces production of cholesterol by the liver.

Another way probiotics bring down cholesterol levels is that as bacteria grow in the intestinal tract, they consume some of the cholesterol that is present, incorporating it into their own cells. This means the cholesterol becomes unavailable for absorption from the intestine into the blood stream, naturally lowering total cholesterol.[43]

I love all the things good bacteria do!

Irritable Bowel Syndrome

Irritable bowel syndrome (IBS) is frequently diagnosed in the young and the old, and it's usually identified by a group of symptoms: abdominal pain, bloating, and a change in movement that can alternate between diarrhea and constipation. My daughter Maci received this diagnosis on the basis of her symptoms of abdominal pain with frequent diarrhea or constipation. Medical treatments seem to do little to help, and so I started looking for an alternative. It was cultured foods and prebiotics that set her free from this debilitating condition by creating a new microbiome in her gut.

So what do scientists say about the connection between probiotics, a healthy gut, and IBS?

One 2014 study looked at 28 people suffering from IBS. Some of the participants were asked to consume a fermented milk product for four weeks, while others served as a control group. In those people consuming the drink, researchers saw an increase in the bacteria that produces butyrate, an acid that is beneficial for gut health. In response, the symptoms of their IBS also improved, while the symptoms of the people in the control group remained.[44] The conclusions drawn in this study mirror those of a study done in 2009 with 34 participants.[45]

Another interesting study, which was done in Norway, compared three groups: two composed of people who were suffering from IBS and one with subjects who had no symptoms of IBS. One of the IBS groups was given dietary advice, and the other two groups didn't receive this advice. Many people who have IBS avoid dairy because it causes their symptoms to flare up. The people in the IBS group who got advice were told to consume fermented milk products containing probiotics. Interestingly the people who consumed the most fermented dairy did significantly better than their counterparts. They reported an improvement in quality of life and a reduction of abdominal pain.[46]

It is exciting to see that doctors are starting to prescribe probiotics as a standard treatment for IBS, but adding fermented foods to each meal can also go a long way in restoring the gut. My daughter had a small portion of cultured food at every meal—kefir for breakfast, a side of cultured veggies and kombucha for lunch and dinner—and ate real, whole foods. This allowed the bad pathogens to be overtaken by the good microbes and allowed her gut lining to heal.

Kidneys/Kidney Stones

There is currently a surge in the use of probiotics for kidney health in the medical field. New probiotic supplements have been developed specifically to treat the kidneys, and there have been remarkable results. Certain strains of probiotics can gobble up urea, uric acid, creatinine, and many other toxins that are not being eliminated by underperforming kidneys. As the healthy bacteria grow and multiply, they consume more and more of these poisonous substances, reducing the serum uremic toxin levels in people with compromised kidney function.[47] Here's one of my favorite stories about cultured foods and kidney health:

> I wrote to you a couple of months ago desperate for some help. My kidney doctor had just told me that my kidneys were functioning at 20 percent and I needed

to choose which form of dialysis I would prefer. It was a death sentence to me. I have had several health problems through the years, and this was heading for a crash really soon! I had asked you if you had ever heard of anyone who had tried this cultured-food-and-drink way of life with any results of repairing kidney function, and you told me not that you had heard of, but you gave me encouragement to try it anyway. In my grief and despair I decided to do just that. Donna, I went back to the kidney care doctor just recently and he just kept shaking his head and said he didn't understand how or why this way worked, but that not only had I lost weight in the two months since I last saw him, but also my kidney function . . . went UP 10 percent!!!!! Yay God! He said he had never heard of this happening before. The nurse came back in after the visit and said in all the years she had worked for him she had never seen him speechless like that. All this, Donna, after only doing it for approximately 1½ months!

Not only are people seeing improvement in kidney function, but they are also seeing that cultured foods can help prevent kidney stones.

A kidney stone is a solid piece of material that forms in the urinary tract when there are high levels of certain substances in the urine. For about 80 percent of Americans who have kidney stones, this substance is calcium oxalate. While this is naturally found in urine, calcium oxalate and the other substances found in kidney stones do not normally cause problems, because they are at a relatively low concentration. They usually pass through the body and are disposed of in urine. However, when they reach high concentrations, the body isn't able to pass all of them, so they form into kidney stones. There are many ways to treat kidney stones, including surgical removal or the use of shock waves to break up the stones into smaller, passable pieces, but these treatments don't address why they develop in the first place.

There is one bacterium naturally found in the digestive tract, *Oxalobacter formigenes*, that has been shown to degrade calcium oxalate, thus preventing kidney stones. Its levels vary depending on gut acidity and salts, and in some individuals it cannot be detected. It is also very susceptible to commonly used antibiotics. In one study, adult volunteers who ingested a dose of *O. formigenes* had a reduced concentration of calcium oxalate in their urine.[48] While it is not known if *O. formigenes* is in cultured foods, another study showed that bacteria strains in cultured foods could be just as effective at reducing calcium oxalate concentrations. This was seen in a four-week study in which six patients with major risks for kidney stones received a daily probiotic containing *L. acidophilus*, *L. plantarum*, *Lactobacillus brevis*, *S. thermophilus*, and *B. infantis*—all of which are found in cultured foods. The results showed a great reduction of calcium oxalates in all six subjects.[49] Another study, done by the California Dairy Research Foundation and Dairy and Food Culture Technologies, got similar results in a study of 10 people.[50]

Isn't it exciting that these foods can make such a difference!

Obesity

Many people have told me that consuming cultured foods has led to weight loss. And it doesn't matter which food—kombucha, kefir, and cultured veggies all seem to give the body the nutrients it needs to feel satiated, which leads to eating less. Incorporating cultured foods also helps you wean yourself from the addictive substances and cravings that leave you in a vicious cycle of unhealthy eating.

So much research has been done about the connection between a healthy weight and a healthy gut that I'm not going to go into it all here. In short, the outcome of many of these studies is that a diverse community of bacteria is important for maintaining a healthy metabolism and weight.

Dr. Raphael Kellman, who founded the Kellman Center for Integrative & Functional Medicine, has written a great book called *The Microbiome Diet,* which sums up the connection between weight and a healthy gut:

> These beneficial bacteria make up a separate ecology within the body and have an enormous influence on your metabolism, your hormones, your cravings— even your genes. . . . When it operates at peak efficiency, so does your metabolism. And when your microbiome is out of balance, you might find yourself gaining weight or unable to lose weight, no matter how much you exercise or how carefully you eat. To achieve your ideal weight, you need the help of your microbiome.[51]

Before I step away from the section on obesity, I do want to zero in on one aspect of the weight-loss journey that many people don't know is associated with a healthy gut: cravings.

In our family we don't have a lot of sugar; mostly we eat things made with healthier sweeteners, such as stevia or Sucanat. But not long ago sugar started to creep back into my life, and I started to feel the effects. It started to change me, and my body let me know by causing intense cravings for sugar. Why does this happen?

It's because different bacterial species need different things to survive. Some like sugar. Some like fat. And when you feed your body sugar or fat, you strengthen the bacteria that feed on these substances, helping them multiply. And with more of them, the need for sugar or fat is greater. Because the gut is linked to the immune system, the endocrine system, and the nervous system, the signals for this increased need are sent to your brain, and this influences your desires and your behavior. By eating the desired substance, you throw off the balance of your gut even more dramatically, causing cravings to intensify. This is what happened to me when I started wanting sugar all the time.

The exciting part is that we have some control in this. We can change the bacterial makeup of our microbiome by changing what we eat. By adding cultured foods and prebiotics (food for bacteria) and by removing highly processed foods and sugar, we cause our bacteria to change; in turn, they change our desire for certain foods. And this decreasing of cravings can start in as little as 24 hours!

Ulcers

Peptic ulcers, which are open sores in the lining of the stomach or upper small intestine, can be very painful. They create a burning sensation in the gut and cause painful gas and nausea, making it difficult to eat. For years no one knew what caused them, but in 2005, scientists Barry Marshall and J. Robin Warren were awarded the Nobel Prize in Physiology or Medicine for their discovery that peptic ulcers were caused primarily by the bacterium *Helicobacter pylori*. Quite a few studies have examined the effects of probiotics on *H. pylori*, and it seems that many different strains of probiotic bacteria have a beneficial effect on lessening the number of *H. pylori* in the gut, thus protecting against ulcers. Scientists haven't yet determined the exact reason for this, but some theorize that it is related to either changing the pH of the stomach, thus inhibiting the growth of *H. pylori*, or preventing *H. pylori* from adhering to the stomach's membrane.[52] Whatever the reason, it seems that the addition of probiotic foods to the diet helps prevent *H. pylori* from wreaking havoc on the gut.

One study looked at the issue of ulcers from another angle and found a decreased risk for ulcers in people who had a high intake of fermented milk products. An increased risk was noted for high milk intake.[53]

Another study found that adding lots of prebiotic foods to your diet may help prevent stomach ulcers. This study observed nearly 48,000 men between the ages of 40 and 70 for six years and analyzed their eating habits. It was found that men with the highest intake of soluble fiber substantially reduced their risk of developing an ulcer.[54]

Among people who already have ulcers, kombucha has been found to help the healing process. The special probiotic bacteria and yeasts in kombucha protect the lining of the gut by reducing the acids that damage the mucous membrane. It was found that this works as well as the prescription drug Prilosec in healing stomach ulcers.[55]

Cultured vegetables have a part in healing ulcers as well. Vitamin U, which is not actually a vitamin but a compound called S-methylmethionine, is abundant in cultured cabbage and its juices and has been shown to successfully treat ulcerative colitis, acid reflux, and peptic ulcers.[56]

Yeast Infections

Candida is a yeast/fungal organism that lives naturally within the human body. You can't get rid of it completely, nor should you want to. It helps keep you healthy by recognizing and destroying harmful bacteria. It also digests and breaks down necrotic (dead) material in your body in order to get rid of it. Debris that's too toxic or difficult for our regular digestive system can be handled by candida. But when it overgrows and gets out of control, problems arise. One of the faster ways for candida to get out of control is to take antibiotics. A balance of good bacteria keeps candida in check. A common practice among researchers looking to induce a yeast infection is actually to give subjects antibiotics to purposely throw off the balance of their microbiomes.

Overproduction of candida can cause many illnesses, including the fungal infection candidiasis. Candida can spread throughout the intestines and sinuses, and if it goes systemic, it can penetrate the bloodstream, releasing toxic by-products.

In women, bacteria normally colonize the vagina and keep candida and yeast infections under control. There are five known vaginal bacteria, and many of them, like *Lactobacillus,* produce lactic acid, which lowers the pH, creating a hostile environment for pathogens. When these bacteria are killed by things such as antibiotics, an overgrowth of yeast may result, leading to a yeast infection.

A lot of people avoid cultured foods—especially kombucha—when they have an overgrowth of candida, believing that these foods actually make the condition worse. As I noted in the last chapter, this isn't what I've found to be true. In fact, it's just the opposite: cultured foods can aid in the treatment of candida overgrowth, as long as they are made properly in order to remove the sugars and allow the probiotics to grow and become strong.

There are now some studies supporting my life experiences. One study included 150 hospitalized children (106 boys, 44 girls) between the ages of 3 months and 12 years who had been on broad-spectrum antibiotics for at least 48 hours. They were divided into one trial group and one placebo group. For seven days, the subjects in the trial group received a sachet of probiotics twice a day; the other group received placebo packets. Each probiotic sachet contained *Lactobacillus acidophilus, Lactobacillus rhamnosus, Bifidobacterium longum, Bifidobacterium bifidum, Saccharomyces boulardii* (the good yeast in kombucha), and *Saccharomyces thermophilus*—all of which are common in cultured foods—and fructo-oligosaccharides, which are a type of prebiotic.

The presence of candida was the same in both groups on the first day, but on the last day that probiotics were administered, 27.9 percent of the patients in the trial group were colonized with a candida infection, compared with the 42.6 percent of the patients in the placebo group. Candida infections continued to increase in number from day 7 to day 14 in the placebo group but not in the one that took the probiotic sachets. This showed that supplementing with probiotics could help reduce candida colonization in critically ill children receiving broad-spectrum antibiotics.[57]

Other studies show that when you add probiotics from the *Lactobacillus* family you down-regulate candida, stopping yeast infections and keeping them from recurring.[58] I can think of no better way to do this than through cultured foods, which are loaded with many probiotics, especially those from the *Lactobacillus* family.

Bringing It All Together

Now you know some of the wonderful ways that bacteria are helping us stay healthy and happy. Research is popping up left and right to support the benefits of bacteria, and every week I hear firsthand stories of healing from people on my website and in my classes.

It's amazing what probiotic foods can do. And it's surprising that something so simple can help you with all sorts of symptoms. Are you constipated? Try cultured foods. Are you having the opposite problem? Try cultured foods. Do you feel tired and run-down? Just start with one cultured food and give it a try. You are what you eat, after all.

When I was sick, I never realized how good I could feel. Even when I wasn't sick, I didn't know that I could feel better. But when I started eating cultured foods, my emotions changed from despair to joy. My body did a complete turnaround, and so did my life. Never in a million years did I think that I would have the life I have now. Write a book? No way! Have a website and online store and teach classes helping thousands of people? That wasn't even a possibility to me. But when I began to feel better, I found special gifts and talents I never knew I had. As my body healed, it opened up my heart, and all I wanted to do was help others feel the same. We really are made to help one another. It's a desire that I think we are born with. What gifts and talents do you have that you don't know about because you don't feel good? Don't spend your life not feeling good. You don't know what you're missing. You have a hundred trillion friends who want to see you well, and one more friend who wants to help you, too. And that friend is me. So now let's get with the program and learn the practicalities of bringing cultured foods into your life.

CHAPTER 5

Bringing the Trilogy into Your Life

"It is our choices that show what we truly are, far more than our abilities."

—Albus Dumbledore

A habit is something you do pretty much automatically. Once you realize you are doing it, you can stop or decide to continue. At that point it becomes a choice, not a habit. So why do we continue to do things that bring negative consequences into our lives even when we realize that we can choose? Perplexing, isn't it? We all know that we will feel better if we eat better. I hear this all the time, and I said it to myself for many years. Still I continued to make choices that hurt me instead of benefited me. Why? It took me a long time to figure this out. Maybe my little revelation will help clear the cobwebs of confusion for you.

Every time we make a choice about anything, but especially about what we eat, we are making that choice because in that moment we believe it will benefit us. Now hold on—I know what you're thinking: *"This is not true. I often eat food that I know isn't good for me."* You may very well know it's not good for you, but *in the moment* there is a reason you are choosing it. I did this for years. In the short term, I chose what I felt I needed. I was too tired to fix a healthy meal, so I went for something quick and easy. I was craving comfort, so ice cream sounded good. Often when I made these choices I would think, *I will just do this tonight, and tomorrow I will start anew.*

These short-term choices went on and on until my family and I got sick. Then it became clear that something needed to change. When my children started to suffer because of my choices, I couldn't stand the pain. So I changed, mostly for them, but in turn it healed me, too. At first it felt like an uphill battle, but in the end it set me free. Like so many others, I had been trained to think that eating healthy is hard. But I found out that this isn't true.

Keep in mind, I didn't change all at once. I went one small, fermented step at a time. And as I made good choices, my healthy life picked up momentum. Every good choice I made led to more good choices, and before I knew it my family and I were getting better. I felt so good that I never looked back.

Making these choices rewired my brain and changed the world of bacteria inside of me. It made me realize that what I really wanted was ease and to feel good. My cravings for unhealthy foods subsided, and I started craving the foods that made me thrive.

Now it's time for you to start making your own healthy changes. This is where the fun begins. Don't be intimated. I know this cultured food stuff sounds hard, but I promise it isn't; it's just new. I have made the easiest guide I can think of for you. I've tried to make it fun and feel like an adventure. Before you know it, cultured food will be a normal part of your life, and you'll wonder how you ever lived without it. Once you taste the freedom that health gives you, you will be soaring. When you are well, you will become a beacon to others, and everybody will want to know what you have done to get so healthy. In this way, you'll literally change the world by changing yourself—and your hundred trillion helpers can't wait to help you.

Getting Started

Before we begin, I need to caution you about what you are about to undertake. These are not simply *foods*; they're powerful *medicine*. These foods will flood your body with billions of probiotics.

The ability of these bacteria to heal you depends on their strength and numbers. As you eat more and more of them, along with prebiotics, you will create a powerful healing army. When they gather enough members of their particular strain, they will begin to dominate and change the environment inside your body. This means that they will destroy pathogens and yeasts that have been in control. While this is good news, it can cause symptoms that make you feel as if you're getting worse, not better. But these are temporary.

This is called a healing crisis, or if you'd like to go by the medical term, a Herxheimer reaction, and it is just the first stop on the road to recovery. The reason symptoms occur is that when harmful bacteria and yeasts die, they produce toxins. This can make you feel pretty bad if you have a lot of them and your body is not able to eliminate them quickly enough to keep up with the healing process. Some of the symptoms you may notice are:

- Body odor
- Diarrhea or loose stools
- Digestive upset
- Discolored stools
- Fatigue
- Fever
- Gas and bloating
- Headaches
- Hot or cold flashes
- Increased urination
- Joint pain
- Sinus stuffiness or drainage
- Sore throat

The vast majority of people experience very mild symptoms or none at all. Only a few people will experience severe symptoms. How bad you feel depends on the health of your gut when you begin. But the negative effects of eating cultured foods will subside as the body gets healthier and is able to eliminate toxins more effectively. Symptoms usually lessen or end within two to three days, but on rare occasions they can last a few weeks.

My own healing crisis was very brief. When I started consuming cultured foods I experienced a slight fever, which lasted for about an hour and then left. I also had increased urination and fatigue, which lasted a few days. And when they went away I felt a renewed state of being that I had not known before.

So what do you do if these symptoms occur? I suggest that you consume cultured foods more slowly or even take some time off and let your body clear itself. Then begin again after a few days or even a couple of weeks. In short, I suggest you listen to your body. This is one of the greatest tools cultured foods offered me. I learned that my body was sending me messages all the time. It was talking to me in symptoms, but I hadn't thought about it in this way. Directly experiencing the power of cultured foods opened my eyes to this. Now I can't eat the foods that created illness in me. This will happen to you, too, if you just listen to what your body is telling you.

So please don't give up even if you experience negative side effects. This is just your body letting you know that you're on the right path. Go very slowly and see how your body reacts. Add only one cultured food at a time, eating or drinking small amounts of it until your body adjusts and rebalances. Then you can add more.

That being said, I know a few people who decided to take a different approach: they simply flooded their systems with tons of cultured food and good bacteria, waging an all-out war and getting it over with. I had one reader tell me he was going for the nuclear blast instead of the slow, gentle approach. This can be extremely uncomfortable, and it's not for everybody, but it can reestablish the gut more quickly.

One question I get a lot when I start people on the process of eating cultured foods is whether they can get the same effects from taking probiotic supplements, and my answer is a resounding NO. As I mentioned before, probiotics taken in pill form don't make it into the intestine—they are killed by stomach acid. So even though there are billions of healthy bacteria in the pills, these bacteria don't necessarily get where they need to go. But with cultured foods, these bacteria are encased in a protective halo that ushers them through the stomach. The acid attacks the food containing them but doesn't have time to kill the healthy bacteria within. So probiotic foods are much more powerful than their pill counterparts.

TRYING OUT THE TRILOGY

- **Kefir:** Try about ¼ cup the first day and see how you feel. You can try one of my recipes, drink it straight, or sweeten it with a little fruit, honey, or stevia for a sugar-free version. See how you feel, and if you're doing great, you can have some more. If not, let your body adjust. Wait a day or two and try again.

- **Kombucha:** Try about ¼ cup the first day and see how you feel. If you're feeling great, you can have some more. If not, give your body time to adjust. Wait a day or two and try again.

- **Cultured vegetables:** Go slowly and eat only a spoonful per day for the first few days. Pay attention to how you feel. If you're doing great, you can have some more. If not, let your body adjust. Wait a day or two and try again.

I'm so excited for you to begin this journey. Once you experience wellness, the contrast between sick and healthy seems greater, and going back to harmful eating habits becomes harder and harder. Cultured foods changed me for good, and there is no going back. You never know how bad you are actually feeling until you experience how good you're supposed to feel!

Here We Go!

All right! It's time to jump in and start eating! There are a couple of ways to do this. The first is to simply choose which food sounds the best and start. Is it kefir or cultured vegetables? Or does kombucha sound intriguing? There is no wrong choice, so pick one, go to the next chapter ("The Basics"), and start there with the easy, step-by-step instructions. Once you've mastered one food, move to another until you have the whole Trilogy in your diet.

Your other option is to head to the appendix (page 195) and follow the 21-day plan I have outlined. This will take you by the hand and show you exactly how to incorporate all three foods into your diet. It covers everything from shopping to prepping to eating. A lot of people are intimidated by these foods, but there's nothing to be afraid of. It's just new, but that's why I am here to help you.

PART II

The Recipes

CHAPTER 6

The Basics

In this chapter, you'll learn how to make the most basic recipes for each element of the Trilogy—cultured veggies, kefir, and kombucha. I'll take you step-by-step through these processes so you can get some experience and gain the confidence you need to jump wholeheartedly into the recipes in the next chapters. I know this can be a bit intimidating, but believe me—these foods are extremely forgiving in the preparation process. And they're safe. But just to be sure you feel empowered to make them, I've also included quite a few troubleshooting tips and some frequently asked questions for each type of food. So let's get culturing!

Making Basic Kefir

Kefir is the simplest part of the Trilogy to make—and one of the fastest: it takes only 24 hours! So in one day you'll be happily on your way to digestive health. There are *two* ways to make kefir: using kefir starter culture packets and using live grains. I'm going to show you both, but I highly recommend that you use the packets if you're just starting out. This is how I began. It's super easy, and anybody can do it, plus you'll get consistent results again and again.

When making either of these recipes, you can use nearly any type of milk that's available. Whole milk, reduced-fat, nonfat, goat's milk, cow's milk, pasteurized, and homogenized—whatever you choose. However, I think fresh, raw, whole cow's milk makes the most delicious kefir. The only thing I recommend you avoid is ultra-pasteurized or lactose-free milk. These don't provide enough food to keep the bacteria happy. And never use a jar still hot from the dishwasher. Heat and lack of food are the two things that will kill the probiotics in your kefir.

Foolproof Kefir Method with Easy Kefir

Making kefir with culture packets is easier than making yogurt, and there are only a few steps. The starter culture, which consists of freeze-dried kefir grains and comes in powder form, and you basically just add milk. Then you're done! Four packages can make up to 28 gallons of kefir. If you're struggling or feel overwhelmed, this is a great place to start. You can purchase Easy Kefir at www.culturedfoodlife.com/store and also at www.cuttingedge cultures.com. Check out step-by-step pictures detailing the process at: www.culturedfoodlife .com/the-trilogy/kefir/how-to-make-kefir/.

Step 1: Place 4 cups of milk* in a glass jar that can be securely sealed. I like canning jars with plastic lids, but you can use any jar that will close securely.

Step 2: Add one packet of Easy Kefir powder.

Step 3: Securely seal the jar and shake or stir well to combine the ingredients.

Step 4: Leave the jar on your kitchen counter, out of direct sunlight or in a cabinet at room temperature (between 68°F and 72°F), for 18 to 24 hours. If your home is cooler than 72°F, you may have to let it ferment for a bit longer. Cooler than 65 degrees might result in kefir that will not ferment properly.

Step 5: When the milk has thickened and has a distinctive, sour fragrance, your kefir is ready. The final consistency is like drinkable yogurt.

Step 6: Place the kefir in the refrigerator. The fermentation process will continue, but the cold temperature will slow it down. You can keep the kefir in your fridge in a sealed container for many months perfectly preserved. But remember, the longer it's in the refrigerator, the more sour it will become and the fewer probiotics it will have.

* If you avoid dairy products, see my dairy-free section (page 57).

Reculturing Kefir

Kefir made with Easy Kefir culture can be recultured, which basically means that you can use the kefir you made as the culture rather than using a new powder packet. This kefir can be recultured anywhere from two to seven times, with the exact number depending on the freshness of your kefir. I recommend reculturing within seven days of making each batch. Longer periods between batches will decrease the likelihood that the new batch will culture successfully.

Step 1: Place 3¾ cups of milk* in a glass jar that can be securely sealed. I like canning jars with plastic lids, but you can use any jar that will close securely.

Step 2: Add ¼ cup of the kefir from the previous batch.

Step 3: Stir to combine the ingredients, then securely seal the jar. Or you can simply seal the jar and shake it to mix everything together.

Step 4: Leave the jar on your kitchen counter, out of direct sunlight, or in a cabinet at room temperature, for 18 to 24 hours. If your home is cooler than 72°F, you may have to let it ferment for a bit longer.

Step 5: When the milk has thickened and has a distinctive, sour fragrance, your kefir is ready. The final consistency is like drinkable yogurt.

Step 6: Place the kefir in the refrigerator. The fermentation process will continue, but the cold temperature will slow it down. You can keep the kefir in your fridge in a sealed container for many months perfectly preserved. But remember, the longer it's in the refrigerator, the more sour it will become and the fewer probiotics it will have.

Making Kefir with Kefir Grains

Now that I'm more experienced, I use live grains to make my kefir. These grains, which look a bit like cottage cheese, are actually groups of many different strains of beneficial bacteria and yeasts that feed on the lactose in milk. By eating the lactose, they grow and thrive, multiplying and overtaking any bad bacteria. They turn the milk they are in into a probiotic powerhouse.

Making kefir using grains is still really easy, but it's a bit more involved because you have to keep your grains fed and happy. In return they will make you delicious kefir—and they last forever if you take care of them. One of the reasons I changed my culturing method is because kefir made from grains is actually a lot stronger than kefir made from the powder packages.

You can use the method below to make any amount of kefir you desire. The most important thing to remember is to use 1 tablespoon of kefir grains per 3 cups of milk.* So, if you want to make 3 cups of kefir, use 1 tablespoon of kefir grains and 3 cups of milk. For 6 cups of kefir, use 2 tablespoons of kefir grains and 6 cups of milk. And so on.

* If you avoid dairy products, see my dairy-free section (page 57).

Step 1: Place the kefir grains in a glass jar that can be securely sealed, using 1 tablespoon of grains for each 3 cups of kefir you want to make. I like canning jars with plastic lids, but you can use any jar that will close securely.

Step 2: Add the appropriate amount of milk to the jar.

Step 3: Securely seal the jar and leave it on your kitchen counter—out of direct sunlight—or in a cabinet at room temperature for 24 hours.

Step 4: After 24 hours, remove the kefir grains, using a slotted spoon or a mesh strainer. (The strainer can be stainless steel or plastic.) Add the kefir grains to fresh milk to begin another fermentation or for storage (see page 55).

Step 5: Transfer the strained kefir to your refrigerator. At this point it is ready to drink or to start a second fermentation (see page 55). You can keep the kefir in your fridge in a sealed container for many months perfectly preserved, but remember, the longer it's in the refrigerator, the more sour it will become and the fewer probiotics it will have.

Caring for Your Kefir Grains

If you've chosen to use grains to make your kefir, you'll need to tend to them in order to make sure they remain active over the long term. To do this, you have to keep them away from heat and supply them with plenty of food. If you want to take a break from making kefir for more than one or two days—for instance, if you will be away from home—you need to care for your grains in a specific way.

Step 1: Place your kefir grains in fresh milk. Keep in mind the ratio rule of 1 tablespoon of grains to 3 cups of milk.

Step 2: Place this jar of kefir grains and milk in the refrigerator.

With this ratio of grains to milk, the grains will stay alive for one week in the refrigerator. If you are going to be gone for more than one week, simply multiply the amount of milk by the number of weeks you will be away. For example, if you are going to be gone two weeks, double the amount of milk with the grains. Three weeks, triple it.

When you return to making kefir, the milk you drain from the stored kefir grains is not really kefir. You can still drink or use it, but it doesn't taste the same as kefir made on the counter. It's been kept at too low a temperature in the fridge to ferment properly. I usually just discard this milk.

Extracurricular Kefir Activities

Here are some of the extra things I regularly do with kefir. They make my kefir taste better and add variety to recipes.

Second-Fermenting Kefir

Many years ago, I discovered that a second fermentation not only makes kefir taste better, but also increases its nutrients. It is now the only way I make it! Second fermenting isn't difficult, and it reduces some of the sourness. The process also increases certain B vitamins, like folic acid, and makes the calcium and magnesium more bioavailable (meaning that your body can take in more of the nutrients and use them immediately).

Second-fermenting your kefir can be done with almost any fruit or spice. Basically, it entails adding a flavor of your choice to the kefir, sealing the container, and letting it sit at room temperature for 1 to 3 hours—how long you leave it depends on how intense you want the flavor to be and your preferred kefir texture. The longer it second-ferments, the more likely it is to separate into whey and curds. Although this isn't a bad thing, some people like kefir better when it stays creamy. If you want creamier kefir, second-ferment it outside the fridge for only an hour and then transfer it to the refrigerator. The cold will slow the fermentation while allowing the flavor of your fruit or spice to intensify.

I have second-fermented my kefir using all sorts of flavorings, from cinnamon sticks and orange or lemon peel to chai tea and strawberries and blueberries. To get the intensity of flavor you want, it often takes some experimentation. For example, when I first used a chai tea bag, I let it ferment for 3 hours; the chai flavor ended up being too strong, so on the next batch I left it at room temperature for only 1 hour, and it was perfect! For second-fermenting with fruit, I generally recommend that you use one or two pieces of small fruit, such as strawberries, or ⅛ cup of chopped fruit for the first attempt. You can use more or less in the next batch, depending on how you like it. You can even use just the peel of the fruit for wonderful flavor. If you'd like to learn more about some of the flavors I've come up with, you can check out my post about second-fermented kefirs at www.culturedfoodlife.com/the-trilogy/kefir/how-to-second-ferment-kefir.

Here is a recipe for one of my favorite second-fermented flavors.

SECOND-FERMENTED CITRUS KEFIR

2 cups Basic Kefir (page 51)

1 organic orange or lemon

Step 1: Place the kefir in a glass jar that can be securely sealed.

Step 2: Using a vegetable peeler, peel one strip of zest from the orange or lemon—the equivalent of one time around the fruit. Avoid the white pith, which is bitter.

Step 3: Place the zest in the jar with the kefir and close securely.

Step 4: Leave the jar on your kitchen counter, out of direct sunlight, for 1 to 3 hours to ferment a second time.

Step 5: After 1 to 3 hours, transfer the jar to the refrigerator, leaving in the zest. This kefir can be stored in the fridge in its jar for one year.

Making Kefir Cheese and Whey

Making kefir cheese is one of my favorite things to do with kefir. I make it regularly and use it almost every day. It is a great substitute for cream cheese or sour cream in any recipe, and it's super easy to make. You can also use the whey to make cultured vegetables. Check out chapter 10 for many of these recipes. I have no doubt that you'll soon love these as much as I do.

KEFIR CHEESE AND KEFIR WHEY

Makes 1 cup kefir cheese and 1 cup kefir whey

2 cups Basic Kefir (page 51) or Nondairy Kefir (page 57)

....

Step 1: Place a basket-style coffee filter in a strainer and set the strainer over a bowl.

Step 2: Pour the kefir into the coffee filter. Cover the bowl with plastic wrap and place it in the refrigerator overnight. The bowl will catch the liquid whey, which you can store for future use. The next day you'll have a beautiful chunk of kefir cheese. If you would like firmer cheese, you can let the whey continue to drain for a full day or longer.

Storage note: The kefir cheese and kefir whey can be stored separately in airtight containers in the refrigerator for up to 1 month.

Nondairy Kefir Options

Almond-, cashew-, or coconut-milk kefir is a great alternative to dairy kefir if you are avoiding dairy for any reason. These kefirs have benefits similar to those of dairy kefir, though the amounts of calcium and magnesium can differ depending on which milk you use. The probiotic content is just as high, and they are supercharged with vitamins. Interestingly, they also can help people alleviate dairy allergies—I've heard many stories of people whose dairy allergies went away after they drank nondairy kefir for a while.

Using kefir powder packets does not work very well for making nondairy kefir, so I recommend using kefir grains. There is one major difference in the care of kefir grains when you are making dairy-free kefir. Because these grains grow and thrive by eating the lactose in dairy milk, putting them in a lactose-free (nondairy) environment will eventually kill them. However, I have found two ways to keep them thriving for quite a long time:

Method 1: Refresh Your Grains in Dairy. The basic idea here is to put the grains in dairy milk once a week (or more) in order to give them the food they need to live. To do this, simply put the grains in a few cups of milk and let them eat the lactose out of it (in other words, make dairy kefir). Then you can reuse them to make nondairy kefir again. The more often you do this, the more your grains will grow and multiply. You can rinse the grains in coconut or almond milk to remove the dairy if you are allergic.

Method 2: Feed Your Grains Date Paste. In this method, you simply make a paste from dates and add a little to the nondairy milk each time you make kefir. (See specific steps on page 54.) This provides your grains with a source of fuel to keep them alive and thriving. To make date paste:

1. Cover 12 whole, pitted dates with water and let them soak until they're soft, about 3 to 4 hours.

2. Drain the dates, reserving the soaking water.

3. Place the dates in a food processor or blender. Process them, adding the soaking liquid 1 tablespoon at a time, until the mixture is smooth but still thick. This will require ¼ to ½ cup of the soaking water, depending on the type, freshness, and softness of the dates.

4. Place the paste in a jar with a secure lid and store in the fridge.

Another option is to use your kefir grains exclusively to make nondairy kefir and accept that they won't live forever. They should last many months this way, but you'll need to purchase more grains when they stop making kefir.

BASIC ALMOND-, CASHEW-, OR COCONUT-MILK KEFIR

You can use the method below to make any amount of kefir you desire. Use the same ratio of grains to milk as for dairy kefir: 1 tablespoon of kefir grains per 3 cups of milk. So if you want to make 3 cups of kefir, use 1 tablespoon of kefir grains and 3 cups of milk. For 6 cups of kefir, use 2 tablespoons of kefir grains and 6 cups of milk. And so on.

Step 1: Place the desired amount of unsweetened nondairy milk into a glass jar that can be securely sealed. I like canning jars with plastic lids, but you can use any jar that will close securely. If you are using date paste, stir it in now. You will use ¼ teaspoon of date paste for each cup of milk. Simply mix it into the milk with a spoon.

Step 2: Add the appropriate amount of kefir grains to the jar, using 1 tablespoon for each cup of milk.

Step 3: Securely seal the jar, and leave the jar on your kitchen counter—out of direct sunlight—or in a cabinet at room temperature for 18 to 24 hours. Almond or coconut milk will culture faster than dairy milk.

Step 4: After 18 to 24 hours, remove the kefir grains by using a slotted spoon or a mesh strainer. (The strainer can be stainless steel or plastic.) Add the kefir grains to fresh almond or coconut milk to begin another fermentation.

Remember to refresh the grains each week by making dairy kefir or by using date paste in your kefir-making process. And if you are going to store the grains or take a break from making kefir, it is best to store them in whole dairy milk or add some date paste as a source of fuel. Follow the instructions for storing kefir grains on page 54.

Frequently Asked Questions about Kefir

Why is my kefir starting to separate and curdle?

It has cultured faster than expected. This is not a bad thing. It just means that your kefir is ready. Remove the grains if you're using them, and then shake or stir the kefir to mix it together again. Or, if you want to make it really creamy, add a small scoop of the prebiotic Prebio Plus. Shake it up, then place the overfermented kefir (grains removed) in a blender and mix for a few seconds. Then place it in a jar in the fridge and let it sit for 8 hours.

Why is my kefir culturing so fast, and how do I fix it?

This happens for one of two reasons: If you're using grains, it's possible that your grains have grown but the amount of milk you're using hasn't increased. Or your kitchen is too warm.

If the former, either remove some of the grains or add more milk for the next batch so the grains-to-milk ratio remains correct. If a too-cozy kitchen is the problem, reduce the amount of time that you leave the kefir out to culture.

I left my kefir grains in the refrigerator for a few months. Are they still good?

Probably not. Kefir grains eat the milk sugars (lactose) out of the milk to live and to make their bacteria. This is why the milk gets more sour over time. When the grains run out of food, they begin to die. They're living organisms and need food. Treat them like a pet and make sure you feed them.

I stored my kefir grains in the fridge for a week. Is the milk that the grains were stored in okay to drink?

The milk that the grains were stored in is not really kefir. It won't hurt you to drink it, but it probably won't taste very good. Milk needs to culture at a warmer temperature to turn into kefir.

Do I culture kefir with a lid or with cheesecloth?

I always culture my kefir with a lid on. I use a one-quart glass canning jar with a plastic lid, but a metal lid is also fine.

Why aren't my kefir grains growing?

If you are making kefir every day, your grains should be growing and multiplying. If they aren't, it is because the temperature in your house is cooler than 68 degrees, which slows down the grains, or your kefir grains have died. If your milk is turning into kefir by becoming sour and thick, your grains are still working, just at a slower rate. You can purchase more or get some new grains from a friend.

How do I know if my kefir grains are still good?

They will culture your milk and turn it sour and thick usually within 24 hours. Make sure that you have enough grains for the amount of milk that you are using.

Making Basic Kombucha

Making your own kombucha may seem a little scary at first, but I assure you it's quite easy. One of the things I recommend to most people before they try making it at home is to buy a bottle of kombucha at the health food store. There are many brands and flavors, and by trying one you'll not only see how delicious it is but get a feel for how it is supposed to look and taste.

Once you've decided to make your own kombucha, you'll have to gather the necessary supplies:

- One-gallon glass jug or non-lead-based crock
- Breathable cloth napkin that will fit completely over the top of the jug or crock
- Rubber band to go around the neck of the jug or crock
- Starter

When I say *starter*, I mean that you will need a kombucha SCOBY (that is, a "symbiotic culture of bacteria and yeast") and one cup of brewed kombucha tea. If you have a friend who makes kombucha, he or she probably has a SCOBY to spare. There is also a worldwide sharing group where you can find people who are willing to share their cultures (www.kefirhood.com). Otherwise, you can buy a starter kit online. I offer them in my store (www.culturedfoodlife.com/store), or you can get them from Wise Choice Market (www.wisechoicemarket.com). Whatever kit you get should come with one SCOBY and one cup of fermented tea. I don't recommend getting a dehydrated SCOBY, as these don't work as well.

I'd like to make a comment here about sugar. You'll see in the recipe below that I list three types of sugar: Sucanat, white sugar, and coconut sugar. Sucanat is a brand of pure, dried sugarcane juice. Because it is minimally processed, it retains the nutrients that are removed from white sugar in the refining process. It also contains less sucrose than refined sugar. However, it does have a slight maple or barley taste, so it's not for everyone. Most of the time, I use regular white sugar when I make kombucha because I like the way it makes my kombucha taste. Also, the sugar gets eaten and as the good bacteria proliferate, so I don't have to worry that I will consume too much sugar.

One last thing to discuss: the type of tea to use. I've noted in the recipe that you should use black or green tea, but honestly, any type of tea (or combination of teas) will work. You just have to figure out which one you like best. Do, however, avoid herbal teas or fruit-flavored teas with oils, as they have antibacterial qualities that could affect the outcome of your kombucha.

BASIC KOMBUCHA

A note before you begin: At the end of this process, you will have created your very own SCOBY. Make sure to keep this—plus one cup of the kombucha you've made—to use as the starter for your next batch.

Makes 3 quarts

3 quarts filtered water (not distilled)

1 cup Sucanat, white sugar, or coconut sugar

4 or 5 tea bags (organic green tea is preferred, but black tea is good, too)

1 SCOBY

1 cup fermented kombucha tea

Step 1: Wash all utensils with hot, soapy water and rinse well.

Step 2: Bring the filtered water to a boil in a large pot over medium-high heat. When the water has reached a rolling boil, add the sugar and continue to boil for 5 minutes.

Step 3: Turn off the heat and add the tea bags. Steep for 10 to 15 minutes; then remove the tea bags and let the tea cool to room temperature.

Step 4: Pour the cool tea into a 1-gallon container.

Step 5: Add the SCOBY, placing it so that the smooth, shiny surface faces up.

Step 6: Add the fermented kombucha tea.

Step 7: Place the cloth over the opening of the container and secure it with the rubber band. This keeps dust, mold, spores, and vinegar flies out of the fermenting tea.

Step 8: Let the covered container sit undisturbed in a well-ventilated and dark place at a temperature between 65° and 90°F for 6 to 15 days. To keep the temperature stable, a heating belt (brew belt) is highly recommended. You can get this from a local brew store or online. The store on my website (www.culturedfoodlife.com /store) has a link to one on Amazon that I really like.

Step 9: To determine whether the tea is ready, do a taste test every couple of days, starting on the fourth day. The tea should be tart, not sweet. However, it should not be overly sour or vinegary. If the tea is sweet, the sugar hasn't been fully converted. If it tastes like sparkling apple cider, it is ready to drink, unless you want it more tart. If the vinegar taste is too prominent, it's probably fermented a bit too long. It won't hurt you to drink it at this point, but you won't receive as many health benefits because the healthy bacteria die off over time as the food supply is gradually reduced. Your tea should also be a little bubbly if it has not been cultured too long. The good yeast makes naturally occurring carbonation, which dissipates over time. If this happens, the kombucha still has health benefits, but it has more probiotics when it is bubbly.

Step 10: When the tea is brewed to your taste, pour it into good, sturdy glass bottles with clamp-down lids. You can repurpose beer bottles with these lids, such as those from Grolsch, or you can buy new bottles that are specifically designed for brewing. Bottles bought at craft stores aren't as sturdy and may explode. Once the bottles are filled, clamp the lids down and place the bottles in the refrigerator. The tea can be stored there for one year or longer. It will eventually turn to vinegar, which you can use as you would any vinegar. The finished kombucha can be second-fermented with various juices (see pages 55 to 56), but it's also delicious as is.

Remember to save your SCOBY and 1 cup of tea from each batch of kombucha to use as a starter for your next batch. Simply make another pot of tea with sugar and add this to your starter and culture to start the process again.

That's all there is to it. Brewing your own kombucha takes one or two weeks, but in the end you'll have a delicious product that you can be proud of.

Extracurricular Kombucha Activities

Flavoring Your Kombucha

Fruit-flavored kombucha is taking the beverage market by storm. A friend of mine visited the tropical island of St. Martin and said she even found it in stores there. Since it's so good for you and fun to make, I completely understand why everyone is clamoring for it. We served bottles of fruit-flavored kombucha at my daughter's wedding reception. A wedding in my family wouldn't be complete without it. Kombucha is family, too!

SECOND-FERMENTED KOMBUCHA

A note before you begin: Make sure you use good, sturdy bottles with clamp-down lids when making this recipe. You can repurpose beer bottles with these lids, such as those from Grolsch, or you can buy new, thick-glass bottles that are specifically designed for brewing. Bottles bought at craft stores aren't as sturdy and may explode.

Makes 3 quarts; 12 servings

Step 1: Mix together one recipe of Basic Kombucha (page 62) and 2 cups of 100 percent fruit juice (any flavor).

Step 2: Transfer the mixture into clean bottles, leaving about 2 inches of space at the top of each. You can strain the mixture through a coffee filter to help prevent another SCOBY from forming.

Step 3: Clamp the bottles shut and date them, so you know when the second fermentation began.

Step 4: Let the kombucha sit in a dark place at room temperature for 1 to 3 weeks.

Step 5: Check the kombucha after each week to see if it is bubbly enough for you. If not, let it ferment longer.

Step 6: Once ready, transfer the bottles to the fridge.

Storage note: This kombucha will last in the sealed container in the fridge for a year but will turn to vinegar over time. It is still fine to drink but might be better used as vinegar because of the sour taste. Once open, the carbonation will start to decrease—just like regular store-bought soda.

Frequently Asked Questions about Kombucha

My SCOBY sank to the bottom when I made my kombucha. Is it okay?

It is 100 percent okay if your SCOBY sinks. Sink or float—it makes no difference to your kombucha. It won't affect the brew or the taste.

My kombucha is still sweet. What did I do wrong?

Your house is probably on the cooler end of the spectrum, and kombucha takes longer to ferment at lower temperatures. Just leave it to ferment longer. I use a brew belt for a dependable temperature. You can also use a heating pad, but brew belts provide a consistent temperature that is more easily controlled than that of a heating pad.

There are some weird, brown stringy things in my kombucha. Is that okay?

Absolutely. You may also see dark-brown spots. Both of these are normal. They're simply a by-product of the good yeasts eating the sugar out of your tea.

What about that clear film that's forming at the top of my jar?

Don't be alarmed! This is your new SCOBY forming! It will grow to the diameter of the jar or crock it is in. So if you have a wide jar, you will have a big SCOBY each time you make kombucha.

What do I do with all these SCOBYs?

Ahhh, the eternal question. Since you grow a new SCOBY each time you make kombucha, you'll have to get creative. The SCOBYs can stack on top of each other and form a SCOBY hotel. I've fed them to a friend's chickens, used them as fertilizer in my garden, given them away—the list goes on and on.

There is mold on my SCOBY. Is it still safe to consume the tea?

No, it's not safe! Throw the tea and the SCOBY out immediately. As for why this happened, there are a couple of possibilities. Sometimes people do not follow the recipe exactly, throwing off the ratio between the ingredients, which in turn throws off the fermentation process. Be exact in your measurements. The other cause can be airborne molds in your home. A few people I know developed this problem because of a leaky roof or because they placed their pot of kombucha in a closet that had poor air circulation.

My tea has a terrible odor. Is it safe to drink?

Your kombucha should have a neutral odor at first, and then gradually take on a more vinegary smell. If you begin to notice a rotten or unpleasant odor, toss the liquid, and carefully examine the SCOBY for any signs of mold. If the SCOBY has no mold, simply start again with fresh, filtered water and starter tea. If there is mold on the SCOBY, toss everything and start again with all new ingredients.

How should I store my SCOBY?

Simply keep it in a jar with a lid and your starter tea (from the previous batch) on your counter for up to a month.

How long will my SCOBY last?

The SCOBY will last a long time but not forever. If it turns black or starts to develop mold, or if it stops culturing your tea, it's time to toss it.

Is it okay to test my kombucha while it's fermenting?

Yes! Feel free to check on it every so often to see how it's doing. To do this, just pour off a couple ounces for a taste test. Such a test might go like this:

- **4 to 6 days**—*Too sweet; not all sugar converted.*
- **7 to 9 days**—*Tastes like sparkling apple cider.*
- **10+ days**—*Vinegar taste becomes prominent.*

Remember to cover it back up after checking it!

Can I cut up my SCOBY?

Yes, absolutely. You need only part of the SCOBY to ferment the tea. You can even make a pot of kombucha without the SCOBY and just use the starter tea. It will take up to three weeks, but it can be done.

How do I increase the carbonation of my kombucha tea?

One of the reasons your kombucha may not be bubbly is because it's fermented for too long. The good yeasts in kombucha eat the sugar and then release carbon dioxide. This is what creates carbonation. If you let it ferment too long, the kombucha goes flat. If you don't let it get vinegary, it will stay bubbly. Second-fermenting is another way to achieve carbonation. The process requires the extra sugars and the juice in the capped-off bottle so the yeast can transform the sugars into natural carbonation.

Making Cultured Vegetables

There are three basic methods for making cultured vegetables: using no culture, using kefir whey, and using a powdered starter culture. I have my favorite method, but any one of them gets the job done.

No matter the method, you first have to choose a fermenting vessel. There are many types you can use. Regular canning jars and those with clamp-down lids work very well, as does a lead-free crock with a tight-fitting lid. However, my favorite way to make cultured vegetables is in a container with something called an airlock lid. This special lid has a hole in the top and a tube filled with water (an airlock tube) is attached. As your vegetables ferment, the gases being created go up into the airlock and become trapped inside the water. This makes your ferments crisper and tastier. You can find these airlocks in the store on my website (www.culturedfoodlife.com/store) though they are by no means necessary.

After choosing a vessel, you have to decide if you want to use a starter culture. You can certainly make your vegetables without one, but the good bacteria will stay at a higher level for longer if you add a culture. The culture will also increase your body's ability to use and grow these beneficial bacteria inside of you. I've given a quick overview of the three methods below. Once you've decided which method you want to use, the fermentation process for all three is pretty much the same.

Method 1: No Culture

You can make cultured vegetables by simply placing your vegetables in a container and submerging them in water. You must add salt with this method—about 1 teaspoon per 1 quart of vegetables—to inhibit the growth of bad bacteria and to create an environment that is safe.

Method 2: Kefir Whey

This is a great way to use the kefir whey left over from making Kefir Cheese (see page 57). For the best results, make sure to use fresh whey—it should be used within a day or two of separating from the cheese. For this method, use about 2 tablespoons of whey for each quart of vegetables. If you're using kefir whey, you can leave out the salt if you'd like. It's not necessary for safe fermentation as above, but the salt will keep your vegetables crunchy.

Method 3: Powdered Culture Packets

This is my favorite method for making cultured vegetables, and I've found that my students have the most success with this as well. In all the cultured vegetable recipes in this book, you'll see that I've listed the product Cutting Edge Starter Culture. I used to work strictly with Caldwell's Starter Cultures, and they are great. However, since I've gotten more knowledgeable in the science of bacteria, I've partnered with some experts in probiotics and fermentation to create Cutting Edge Cultures, and the results are an even more powerful product. If you choose to use another brand of powdered starter culture, the same measurements will apply.

To make your veggies with a powdered starter culture, you simply have to activate the culture by mixing it with water. You will use about ⅛ teaspoon of Cutting Edge Starter Culture and ¼ cup water per quart of vegetables. Just mix it all together and let the mixture sit for 10 minutes. Generally, I mix the culture and then prep the vegetables while the culture activates. With this method, salt isn't necessary for safety, but it will keep your veggies crunchy.

BASIC CULTURED VEGETABLES

Step 1: Choose a container large enough to hold the veggies—generally a 1-quart, 2-quart, or 1-gallon vessel—that can be securely sealed.

Step 2: Prepare the Cutting Edge Starter Culture, if using:

- **For 1 quart:** ⅛ teaspoon Cutting Edge Starter Culture plus ¼ cup water.

- **For 2 quarts:** ¼ teaspoon Cutting Edge Starter Culture plus ½ cup water.

- **For 1 gallon:** 1 packet Cutting Edge Starter Culture plus 1 cup water.

Step 3: Prepare the vegetables.

Step 4: Pack the vegetables and salt, if using, in the container.

Step 5: Add the culture, if using—prepared Cutting Edge Starter Culture or kefir whey—and fill the container with filtered water, leaving at least 2 inches of headspace at the top to let the vegetables bubble and expand as they ferment.

Step 6: Seal the container and let it sit on your kitchen counter, out of direct sunlight, for 6 days.

Step 7: Check the vegetables every day to make sure they are fully submerged. If they have risen above the water, simply push them down so they are fully covered again. If any white spots or coating form, don't be alarmed. This is not mold but a yeast called kahm yeast, and it can form when the veggies being cultured aren't fresh or have risen above the water. It also appears more often if you don't use a starter culture. The yeast isn't harmful, so just scoop it out along with any vegetables it's on and push the rest back under the water.

Step 8: After 6 days, place the vegetables in the refrigerator, where they can be stored for up to 9 months.

You can use this process with any of the three methods listed above, but I find that the no-culture method works well only for sauerkrauts. Feel free to play with different vegetables and spices. I've included quite a few recipes for my favorite cultured veggies in this book. But once you get the hang of culturing, I'm sure you'll start creating your own masterpieces.

Frequently Asked Questions about Cultured Vegetables

My vegetables are rising in the jar. Is this okay?

Yes, this is perfectly normal and expected. Fermented vegetables should rise and expand as they culture, and you'll find that they can often be very bubbly. This is a normal part of fermentation.

Can cultured vegetables develop botulism?

No. Botulism is an issue with canned goods because the heat used in canning kills all the good bacteria. When culturing foods, the healthy bacteria thrive and make it impossible for the bacteria that cause botulism to survive.

How long do I culture my vegetables on the kitchen counter? Can I leave them longer?

For most vegetables, culturing takes six days at room temperature. There are a few vegetables that will culture in only two or three days, and these shorter times are indicated in the specific recipes. If you culture the vegetables longer than six days, they can get too yeasty; the flavor will change, and not for the better. They will also lose some of their probiotics. However, the veggies still have benefits and are safe to eat. The vegetables will continue to ferment after you place them in the fridge, but at a slower rate. The flavors develop and age like a fine wine!

How long can I store my cultured veggies?

In the refrigerator, cultured veggies will keep for up to nine months, and sometimes longer. They continue to ferment but at a much slower rate. I find that many of my vegetables taste better after six weeks in the fridge. It's fun to taste your vegetables at different stages to find out when you like them best.

Why aren't my vegetables crunchy?

Salt is the key. Vegetables without salt become soft and slimy. Vegetables made with salt will stay crunchy.

Can these foods be stored out of the fridge after they have been fermented?

Technically, cultured vegetables can be stored in a cooler basement or cold cellar. However, they will continue to ferment, and in short order they won't taste very good. Cultured veggies do best and taste best at the colder temperatures of a refrigerator.

How will I know if my vegetables are properly fermented?

They will taste sour and the liquid they are in will look bubbly. If your culturing has gone wrong, you will know this by the strong, unappetizing odor the veggies will give off.

What are the white spots on my veggies?

This is one of the things that people find most troublesome. While these appear to be mold, they are actually something called kahm yeast. This yeast is not harmful, but it can look scary and unpleasant and even smell a little strong. It should be removed from the jar only to prevent it from imparting a strong odor or unpleasant taste to the whole batch. If you can't remove it all, don't worry; it won't hurt you.

Not using the freshest vegetables seems to be one of the fastest ways for kahm yeast to appear. I noticed it most when I used cucumbers and carrots that had been sitting in my fridge for a while.

What do I do if the liquid is leaking from the jar while my veggies culture?

This liquid is called the brine, and if you made your jar too full, the brine might leak out. Not a big deal. Simply open the jar, push the veggies down so they are fully covered, and remove a little bit of the liquid or some of the veggies.

CHAPTER 7

Breakfast Treats and Smoothies

CHAI KEFIR SMOOTHIE

I can't tell you how much I love this smoothie. Chai tea has been around for centuries, and I suspect that's because it not only is delicious but also has so many wonderful health-promoting qualities. To make this smoothie, I do something a bit out of the ordinary: I add the contents of a tea bag—not brewed tea—to the smoothie. The flavor it gives this drink is incredible! And the antioxidants you get will make you feel great.

Makes 1 serving

1¼ cups Basic Kefir (page 51)

½ cup unsweetened almond milk

1 teaspoon loose-leaf chai tea or contents of 1 chai tea bag

3 tablespoons pumpkin puree

1 teaspoon vanilla extract

½ teaspoon pumpkin pie spice

2 frozen bananas*

Cinnamon (optional)

Place the kefir, almond milk, chai tea, pumpkin puree, vanilla, and pumpkin pie spice in a blender and mix for 30 seconds.

Add the bananas and blend again. This will make the mixture thick, creamy, and cold, like a milk shake. Garnish with cinnamon, if desired.

*Make sure to peel the bananas before you freeze them!

CASHEW KALE MILK SHAKE

This milk shake is the perfect way to sneak healthy foods into an unsuspecting family member's diet. The cashew kefir makes it creamy and the fruit makes it sweet, so nobody will have a clue that there's kale in this yummy concoction. Except, of course, for the green color. Just tell them it's from a really green banana!

Makes 1 serving

1 cup Cashew Kefir (page 59)

½ cup kale, torn into bite-size pieces

1 frozen banana*

1 teaspoon vanilla extract

1 kiwi, peeled

Stevia or honey to taste

....

Place all the ingredients in a blender and mix at high speed until smooth. Serve immediately.

*Make sure to peel the banana before you freeze it!

HOLIDAY SMOOTHIE

I love mulling spices because they make foods taste like Christmas. Mulling spices include orange peel, which is a prebiotic, and cinnamon and allspice, which have all kinds of anti-inflammatory properties. They also include cloves, which are great for an upset stomach and as an expectorant. Just as we did with the Chai Kefir Smoothie (page 71), we're going to add the contents of a tea bag to enhance the flavor. It's so yummy!

Makes 1 serving

1 cup frozen peach slices

Contents of 1 tea bag of mulling spices

1 tablespoon chia seeds

½ cup Kefir Cheese (page 57)

1 cup unsweetened almond milk

2 tablespoons psyllium husk*

Stevia or maple syrup to taste

Place all the ingredients in a blender and mix at high speed until smooth. Serve immediately.

*Psyllium husk is a prebiotic, so it will feed the healthy bacteria in your gut. Plus it makes your smoothie thicker. But don't count this smoothie out if you can't find this product. It's delicious without it.

VEGGIES AND KEFIR TOAST

This is a superfast breakfast. It takes only a few minutes to whip together, and there are endless options for serving it. My favorite is the combo below, but you can add some extra dill dip or different vegetables to make it your own. It's also good with a drizzle of well-aged balsamic vinegar.

Makes 2 servings

2 tablespoons Creamy Kefir Dill Dip (page 101)

2 slices sprouted, sourdough, or almond bread, toasted

½ cup (total) chopped red pepper, tomatoes, and broccoli

....

Spread the kefir dill dip on the toast. Top with the veggies and serve.

COCO-NUTTY BERRY KEFIR

I can't tell you how many times I ate (and loved!) this recipe while writing this book. I would throw it together, take it outside with my laptop, and sit on a lawn chair and write. Since it was summertime, I used frozen berries to make a cool treat, and as crazy as this may sound, it gave me a lot of inspiration and comfort as I wrote. My husband would laugh at me and say I was glued to the jar in my hand. But as I say, "Never underestimate the power of a mason jar filled with kefir." Just try it—you'll see.

Makes 1 serving

¾ cup Basic Kefir (page 51)

¼ cup shredded coconut

¼ cup chopped pecans

½ cup mixed berries, fresh or frozen

Stevia, honey, or maple syrup to taste

. . . .

Put all the ingredients in a jar or small bowl and mix thoroughly. Serve immediately.

KOMBUCHA COCONUT SMOOTHIE

I've learned over the years that if I want to feel my very best, then kombucha and kefir are a must in the morning. These cultured foods will train you to eat them, and I'm not kidding about that. I never want to go back to the way I used to feel when I was sick and struggling, so it's kefir and kombucha every morning. When I'm in a hurry, I combine them and take them with me in a travel jug. I know it may sound odd, but it's delicious—bubbly, creamy, and utterly filling.

Makes 1 serving

1 banana

1 cup chopped pineapple

3 handfuls spinach

1 cup Coconut Kefir (page 59)

¾ cup Basic Kombucha (page 62)

½ cup ice

....

Place all the ingredients in a blender and process until smooth and creamy.

RASPBERRY KEFIR TOAST

You don't have to eat tons of cultured foods to receive the benefits. A few spoonfuls can make a huge difference because that's all it takes to give the body billions of probiotics. So grab a pot of tea and a slice of this toast and relax, knowing that your body will thank you.

Makes 1 serving

1 slice sprouted, sourdough, or almond bread

1 tablespoon Lemon Kefir Labneh (page 183)

1 tablespoon Fermented Fruit Jam (page 184)

Toast the bread, then spread the labneh and jam on top. Enjoy!

KEFIR EGGS WITH A SIDE OF VEGGIES

These are the fluffiest, lightest, and most delicious eggs I've ever had—and it's because of the kefir I add to them. While the heat does kill the probiotics, you still get many of kefir's beneficial properties, including the heightened vitamin content. Plus the cultured veggies on the side give you your probiotics.

Makes 3 servings

6 pasture-raised eggs

¼ cup Basic Kefir (page 51)

1 teaspoon Celtic Sea Salt

¼ teaspoon fresh ground pepper

1 tablespoon coconut oil

1 tablespoon chopped fresh chives

2 tablespoons crumbled goat cheese

2 tablespoons Cultured Green Tomato Relish (page 186)

Place the eggs, kefir, salt, and pepper in a blender and pulse until the mixture is light and fluffy.

Heat the coconut oil in a skillet over medium-high heat, then pour in the egg mixture.

As the eggs begin to set, gently pull them across the pan with a spatula and fold them over, forming large, soft curds.

Continue cooking—pulling, lifting, and folding the eggs—until they have fully set and no visible liquid remains.

Remove from the heat and top with the goat cheese and chives.

Serve with a side of green tomato relish.

NATURAL-RISE KEFIR CINNAMON ROLLS

This is a great recipe to make when you don't want to use instant yeast in your rolls. Kefir has its own set of natural yeasts that will cause the dough to rise. It also has all sorts of extra minerals and vitamins. Combine these with the healing properties of cinnamon, which include lowering blood sugar and cholesterol and even preventing Alzheimer's disease, and you have one healthy, powerhouse food. Just be sure to buy good organic cinnamon; many commercial cinnamons have a lot of toxins in them. I use Vietnamese cinnamon, which is the strongest, richest, and sweetest variety.

Makes 12 servings

For the cinnamon filling

4 tablespoons unsalted butter, very soft

¼ cup Sucanat

3 teaspoons ground cinnamon

For the cinnamon roll dough

2 ¾ cups sprouted flour

2 tablespoons Sucanat

3 teaspoons baking powder

1 teaspoon salt

3 tablespoons unsalted butter, melted

¾ cup Basic Kefir (page 51)

1 large egg

Flour

½ cup chopped pecans

For the icing

3 tablespoons butter, melted

3 tablespoons maple syrup

2 teaspoons Basic Kefir (page 51)

Preheat the oven to 350°F. Spray a 9 x 13-inch baking pan with nonstick spray.

To make the cinnamon filling, mix all of the filling ingredients in a medium bowl until combined. Set aside.

For the cinnamon roll dough, mix the flour, Sucanat, baking powder, and salt in a medium bowl.

In a separate bowl, whisk together the butter, kefir, and egg.

Add the wet mixture to the dry ingredients and use a wooden spoon to combine until well mixed.

Place the dough on a well-floured surface, sprinkling on more flour as needed to keep the dough from sticking. Roll the dough out into a (roughly) 12 x 8-inch rectangle.

Sprinkle the dough with the cinnamon filling, then the pecans.

Roll up the dough log-style. Cut 1-inch slices and carefully place them flat on the prepared baking pan, leaving a little space between each roll.

Bake the rolls for 20 to 25 minutes, or until they are a nice golden brown. Remove from the oven and allow them to cool while you make the icing.

For the icing, whisk together the icing ingredients in a small bowl until smooth. Spoon icing over the warm rolls and serve.

Storage note: Leftovers can be stored in a covered container in the fridge for 1 week or frozen for up to 1 month.

SUN-FRESH SMOOTHIE

I make this smoothie more than any other for several reasons. First, it is super-duper creamy and thick like pudding. Second, it tastes like summertime because of the fresh basil and lemon juice. And, finally, I make it because it keeps me full for hours. I wrote this entire book sitting outside or on my boat, and I probably had this smoothie 50 times. It just makes me happy.

Makes 1 serving

1 avocado, pitted, with flesh removed from skin

Juice and zest of ½ lemon

4 fresh basil leaves

½ cup Basic Kefir (page 51)

½ cup unsweetened almond milk

½ cup ice

Stevia or honey to taste

....

Place all the ingredients in a blender and mix at high speed until smooth. Serve immediately.

KEFIR PANCAKES

For these pancakes, mix the dry and wet ingredients separately to make them super-light and fluffy and oh so awesome! This recipe works with the science of oils and waters and how you combine them to give you the yummiest pancakes you've ever had. Love them!

Makes 6 pancakes; 3 servings

½ teaspoon baking soda

1 teaspoon baking powder

1 teaspoon Celtic Sea Salt

3 teaspoons Sucanat

2 cups sprouted flour

4 tablespoons butter, melted

2 egg yolks

2 cups Basic Kefir (page 51)

2 egg whites

3 tablespoons Kombucha Strawberry Maple Syrup (page 180)

....

Mix together the baking soda, baking powder, salt, Sucanat, and flour in a large bowl. Set this mixture aside.

Mix the butter and egg yolks together in a small bowl.

Mix the kefir and egg whites together in a medium bowl.

Add the butter mixture to the kefir mixture and stir until combined. Then add this to the bowl of dry ingredients and stir gently to combine.

Heat a lightly oiled griddle or frying pan over medium-high heat.

Pour or scoop the batter onto the griddle, using approximately ¼ cup for each pancake.

Cook until golden brown on each side, approximately 2 minutes per side. Top with the syrup and serve hot.

COCONUT KIWI SUPER SMOOTHIE

This is a potent smoothie that will detox you with huge amounts of vitamin C, coconut oil, and kefir. Coconut has caprylic acid, which is a powerful yeast killer. Kiwi is rich in vitamin C. And the addition of kale and parsley gives you a great start to getting healthy and giving your body what it needs to heal itself.

Makes 2 servings

6 strawberries, hulled

1 kiwi, peeled

1 lime, peeled and segmented

1 large banana

1 large bunch kale

1 handful fresh parsley

1 organic cucumber, cut in chunks

2 tablespoons goji berries

2 tablespoons chia seeds

1 cup Coconut Kefir (page 59)

1 tablespoon coconut oil

1 cup ice

Place all the ingredients in a blender and mix at high speed until smooth. Serve immediately.

OVERNIGHT BLUEBERRY KEFIR OATMEAL

This tastes like blueberry cobbler. It's so good that—even though it's best to let it sit overnight—I usually eat it within a few hours of making it. It's just sitting in my fridge looking at me while it's culturing, and I cannot resist when I see it. This is also great made with blackberries or raspberries.

Makes 1 serving

¾ cup unsweetened almond milk

½ cup Basic Kefir (page 51)

1½ cups blueberries, fresh or frozen

½ cup old-fashioned oats

1 tablespoon chia seeds

¼ teaspoon Celtic Sea Salt

¼ teaspoon cinnamon

½ dropperful (approximately ½ teaspoon) liquid stevia

1 to 2 tablespoons sliced almonds

2 tablespoons shredded coconut

....

Mix together the almond milk, kefir, blueberries, oatmeal, chia seeds, salt, cinnamon, and stevia in a quart-size canning jar.

Cover and refrigerate overnight.

Before eating, top with the nuts and shredded coconut.

This is best eaten within 24 hours of making it.

OVERNIGHT STRAWBERRY KEFIR PUDDING

This is another delicious and easy mason jar recipe. I love these recipes because you throw ingredients in and then wake up to a delightful meal. Plus they look great! The Ball Mason Jar Company makes vintage-style jars in different colors—green, blue, and purple. My husband has taken it upon himself to find me these jars, so I put them to good use all over my home—not just in these scrumptious recipes.

Makes 1 serving

¾ cup unsweetened coconut or almond milk

½ cup Basic Kefir (page 51)

1½ cups chopped strawberries

½ cup old-fashioned oats

1 tablespoon chia seeds

¼ teaspoon Celtic Sea Salt

½ dropperful liquid stevia

Mix everything together in a quart-size canning jar, cover, and refrigerate overnight. This is best eaten within 24 hours of making it.

SHAMROCKIN' SHAKE

This shake will rock your gut flora and your taste buds! When I started using fresh mint in my smoothies, I was blown away by what a difference it made in the flavor. I now have four types of mint growing in my herb garden: chocolate, orange, spearmint, and regular mint. And not only is mint delicious; it contains menthol, which is a natural decongestant that helps break up phlegm and mucus, and it has been used for thousands of years to treat upset stomachs and indigestion. Mint also has an antioxidant called rosmarinic acid, which has been found to relieve seasonal allergies.

Makes 1 serving

½ cup Basic Kefir (page 51)

1½ cups unsweetened coconut milk

1½ cups spinach leaves

½ cup fresh mint leaves

1 large banana

1 cup ice

1 dropperful liquid stevia

Place all the ingredients in a blender and mix at high speed until smooth. Serve immediately.

CHAPTER 8

Dips and Appetizers

KEFIR CHEESE AND VEGGIE TORTE

My family has always loved my kefir and veggie appetizers at the holidays. This is a healthier version and one that gets gobbled up quickly. The flavors are extraordinary. Just look at the ingredients: pistachios, raisins, cranberries, walnuts, kefir, Orangeade Kraut. It's a varied list, but it all tastes great when put together. It's also super pretty.

Makes 6 servings

½ cup shelled pistachios

½ cup raisins

1 tablespoon coconut oil

1 cup Kefir Cheese (page 57)

3 tablespoons Orangeade Kraut (page 137)

2 tablespoons dried cranberries

2 cloves garlic, minced

1 tablespoon finely chopped flat-leaf parsley

1 teaspoon Worcestershire sauce

1 tablespoon Basic Kombucha (page 62)

½ teaspoon Celtic Sea Salt

¼ cup chopped walnuts

Place the pistachios and raisins in a food processor and blend into small pieces.

Add coconut oil and blend again. Press the mixture into the bottom of a 7-inch springform cheesecake pan that is lined with parchment paper. Refrigerate the mixture while you do the next step.

Mix together the kefir cheese, kraut, cranberries, garlic, parsley, Worcestershire, kombucha, and salt in a small bowl. Remove the pistachio and raisin mixture from the refrigerator and pour the kefir cheese mixture on top.

Sprinkle on the walnuts.

Cover the pan with plastic wrap and refrigerate for 3 to 4 hours.

Gently remove the torte from the pan and serve.

KEFIR CHEESE BALL

This is the cheese ball I make during the holidays, and boy, let me tell you—if I don't make it, I never hear the end of it. People love this delicious flavor combination! In fact, they love it so much that I often make two. Once you start serving this at your shindigs, don't be surprised if people begin whining if you don't bring it.

Makes 10 servings

One 8-ounce block cream cheese, softened

1 cup Kefir Cheese (page 57)

2 cloves garlic, quartered

1 teaspoon Worcestershire sauce

½ teaspoon paprika

1 tablespoon minced onion

1 teaspoon Celtic Sea Salt

⅛ cup chopped parsley

1 cup shredded sharp cheddar cheese

1 cup chopped pecans

Place the cream cheese, kefir cheese, garlic, Worcestershire sauce, paprika, onion, salt, and parsley in a food processor. Pulse until well combined.

Add the cheddar cheese and pulse a few more times.

Line a round bowl with plastic wrap and transfer the mixture from the food processor into the bowl.

Wrap the plastic around the cheese mixture, forming it into a ball.

Seal the plastic wrap and place the ball in the refrigerator for about 12 hours to firm up.

Remove the plastic wrap, roll the cheese ball in the pecans, and serve immediately.

LAYERED CULTURED VEGGIES

I don't know what inspired me to make this recipe the first time I did it. Every time I look at it, I think, **This combination of flavors makes no sense.** But I just have to remember that it's delicious. It's one of my favorite things to eat when I'm in a hurry because it's packed with healthy fats and powerful probiotics and fills me up in an instant. But this can also be served as an appetizer or a side dish.

Makes 2 servings

1 avocado, pitted

¼ cup Kefir Cheese (page 57)

¼ cup Orangeade Kraut (page 137)

½ teaspoon black pepper

½ cup Fermented Hummus (page 97)

Handful sprouted corn chips

....

Scoop the avocado flesh out of the skin and chop it into small pieces. Place the pieces in a small bowl.

Mix the kefir cheese and the kraut together; then season with black pepper.

Place the mixture on top of the avocado, and then top with the hummus.

Serve with the sprouted corn chips.

VEGGIE PECAN DIP

This recipe is made with a bunch of different veggies, and the pecans give it tons of flavor. I love serving it as a dip, but it can be used for so many things: You can scoop it into lettuce wraps; or you can mix it with rice, stuff it in tortillas, and top it with tomatoes, lettuce, and kefir cheese. The possibilities are endless!

Makes 4 servings

1 medium portobello mushroom

¼ onion

1 clove garlic

2 cups spinach

5 sun-dried tomatoes

½ cup chopped zucchini

¼ cup Lemon Kraut (page 124)

3 fresh basil leaves

1½ cups pecans

....

Place all the ingredients in a food processor or blender. Depending on the size of your food processor or blender, you may need to work in batches. Process on high speed until fully combined.

Serve immediately or store in the refrigerator. This dip is best eaten within a day.

CULTURED PEACH PICO DE GALLO

We have a peach tree in our yard that, come August, is covered in butterflies and peaches. The butterflies come for the nectar from the fallen peaches, and I leave a few on the ground so they will have food. But the rest I pick up to make delicious dishes like this. When you ferment peaches with tomatoes and fresh cilantro, it adds a zing to salsa you can't get any other way.

Makes 2 quarts; 32 ¼-cup servings

¼ teaspoon Cutting Edge Starter Culture plus ½ cup water, or ¼ cup Kefir Whey (page 57)

2 medium tomatoes

1 medium cucumber

1 medium peach, pitted

1 serrano pepper

¼ cup chopped red onion

¼ cup chopped cilantro

Juice of ¼ lime

2 teaspoons Celtic Sea Salt

1 clove garlic, chopped

If using the starter culture, stir together the culture and the water. Let the mixture sit while you prepare the other ingredients—around 10 minutes.

Chop the tomatoes, cucumber, and peach into small pieces and put them in a large bowl.

Seed the pepper, chop it finely, and add to the bowl along with the onion, cilantro, lime juice, salt, and garlic. Stir to combine.

Transfer the mixture to a 2-quart glass or ceramic container that can be securely sealed.

Add the culture or whey and fill the container with filtered water, leaving 2 inches of headspace to let the vegetables bubble and expand as they ferment.

Seal the container and let it sit on your kitchen counter, out of direct sunlight, for 2 days.

Check the salsa every day to make sure it is fully submerged. If some of it has risen above the water, simply push it down so it is fully covered again. If white spots of yeast have formed on any unsubmerged pieces, do not worry. Remember, this isn't harmful. Just scoop out the yeast and the salsa it's on and push the rest back under the water. (See FAQs on page 69 for more information.)

When the salsa is done fermenting, place it in the refrigerator.

Storage note: The salsa can be stored in an airtight container in the refrigerator for up to 3 months.

KEFIR ORANGE CUPS

This recipe is one of the main reasons I make kefir cheese. I have prepared this recipe so many times it's like my best friend. The combination of oranges and orange zest with a drizzle of honey is to die for. The presentation is beautiful, too!

Makes 1 serving

2 oranges
1 cup Kefir Cheese (page 57)
½ tablespoon honey or ½ dropperful liquid stevia

Zest one orange with a microplane grater and set the zest aside.

Cut both oranges in half and scoop out the flesh carefully with a spoon, leaving the two halves of the nongrated orange peel intact. Set aside the nongrated peel.

Chop the flesh of both oranges into bite-size pieces.

Mix the kefir cheese and orange pieces together in a small bowl and spoon the mixture into the nongrated orange peel halves.

Drizzle with honey or stevia and top with the zest.

PARMESAN CRISPS AND KRAUT

These are great for people with gluten allergies and a quick alternative to store-bought crackers. They take all of 10 minutes to make, including the prep time! If you don't like rosemary, try other seasonings. Paprika adds a smoky flavor, and black pepper can be nice, too.

Makes 10 servings

½ cup shredded or grated Parmesan cheese

1 tablespoon finely chopped fresh rosemary

½ cup Kefir Cheese (page 57)

½ cup Lemon Kraut (page 124)

....

Preheat the oven to 400°F.

Combine the Parmesan cheese and the rosemary in a small bowl.

Spoon a heaping tablespoon of the cheese mixture onto a silicone or parchment-lined baking sheet and lightly pat down. A silicone mat is highly recommended.

Repeat with the remaining cheese, spacing the spoonfuls about ½ inch apart.

Bake for 3 to 5 minutes or until lightly golden and crisp. Leave the crisps on the pan to cool.

Top each Parmesan crisp with a spoonful of kefir cheese and a spoonful of kraut. Serve immediately.

FERMENTED HUMMUS

Hummus is already considered a healthy food, and fermenting it makes it even more nutritious by increasing the availability of the vitamin content and adding probiotics. This hummus becomes predigested, so the body has no trouble assimilating it. Like any cultured food, it becomes supercharged, giving you more energy for your day.

A note before you begin: I recommend sprouted beans in this recipe because sprouting ups the nutritional value a great deal. If you'd like to learn how to sprout, visit www.vegetariantimes.com/blog/how-to-soak-and-sprout-nuts-seeds-grains-and-beans. If you don't have the time or energy to sprout, simply use nonsprouted beans instead. You can use canned beans or other cooked beans.

Makes 6 servings

1 pound cooked garbanzo beans (chickpeas), preferably soaked and sprouted

3 cloves Fermented Garlic (page 181)

6 tablespoons olive oil

4 tablespoons lemon juice

3 tablespoons raw tahini

¼ teaspoon Celtic Sea Salt

1 teaspoon cumin (optional)

1 teaspoon hot curry powder (optional)

1 teaspoon red pepper flakes or Aleppo pepper flakes (optional)

....

Place the beans, garlic, olive oil, and lemon juice in a food processor or blender and pulse until smooth.

Add the tahini and salt and, if using, the cumin, curry powder, and red pepper flakes. Pulse until the hummus is smooth (add more olive oil if necessary).

Serve immediately, or store in an airtight container in the refrigerator for up to 3 weeks.

MEXICAN KEFIR AND SALSA

I don't expect anyone to make complicated recipes, because I don't want to make them either. I live my life simply, and while these foods may take a little time to ferment, once they do you can put them in all kinds of dishes and recipes—fast! This recipe is a perfect example of that. I whip it up in no time and serve it to my family as a snack. It's filling and a little addictive.

Makes 3 servings

1 cup Kefir Cheese (page 57)

½ cup salsa*

1 tablespoon Curtido Salvadoran Kraut (page 133)

3 servings sprouted corn chips

....

Mix the kefir cheese, salsa, and kraut in a small bowl.

Serve immediately with sprouted corn chips.

Storage note: This can also be stored in an airtight container in the refrigerator for up to 3 days.

*Just buy your favorite kind!

VEGGIES LOVE KEFIR CHEESE

This is the way my family most often eats their cultured veggies. We make whole meals from just this dish by serving it with sprouted chips or fresh vegetables. We also eat it when we watch our favorite sports teams on TV. It replaces all the junk food we used to eat and leaves us satisfied and healthy. I can't say enough about this dish; it's become a family tradition.

Makes 1 serving

½ cup Kefir Cheese (page 57)

⅓ cup Orangeade Kraut (page 137)

1 teaspoon fresh cracked pepper

½ teaspoon Celtic Sea Salt

1½ tablespoons toasted sesame seeds

....

Mix together the kefir cheese and kraut. Top with salt and pepper and toasted sesame seeds. Serve immediately, or store in an airtight jar in the refrigerator for up to 3 days.

EARTH AND SUNSHINE DIP

Do you want your picky eaters to eat cultured foods? Then put cultured foods into yummy dips, and they will never know they have just eaten them. This was specifically why I created this dip—and no one was the wiser.

Makes 8 servings

2 cups raw peas

¼ cup freshly squeezed lemon juice

⅛ cup chopped onion

3 cloves garlic, quartered

1 teaspoon cumin

¼ teaspoon red pepper flakes

1½ teaspoons Celtic Sea Salt

¼ cup chopped flat-leaf parsley

1 cup Kefir Cheese (page 57)

3 tablespoons Lemon Kraut (page 124)

3 tablespoons sesame seeds, toasted

Place the peas, lemon juice, onion, garlic, cumin, red pepper flakes, salt, and parsley in a food processor or blender and pulse until smooth.

Add the kefir cheese and pulse a few more times until it is well incorporated.

Place the mixture in a small bowl. Gently stir in the Lemon Kraut and sesame seeds. Serve immediately or store in a covered container in the refrigerator for up to 5 days.

CREAMY KEFIR DILL DIP

This dip is a huge crowd-pleaser. I serve it at parties with carrots, broccoli, and red peppers, and it gets gobbled up in minutes. When there's any left over, which is rare, I spread it on toast and top it with fresh veggies. It's a taste sensation, no matter how you eat it.

Makes 4 servings

½ cup cream cheese, softened

⅜ cup Kefir Cheese (page 57)

2 teaspoons garlic powder

2 tablespoons chopped fresh dill weed or ½ tablespoon dried dill weed

....

Mix all the ingredients together in a small bowl.

Serve immediately or store, covered, in the refrigerator for up to 1 week.

FERMENTED FIESTA DIP

We love Mexican food at our house, and we often make whole meals out of dishes like this. A side of sprouted corn chips and a glass of my Strawberry Kombucha Margarita (page 175) and we have a delicious lunch. But most of the time, I serve this at get-togethers with friends. It's always a hit!

A note before you begin: I recommend sprouted beans in this recipe because sprouting ups the nutritional value a great deal. If you'd like to learn how to sprout, visit www.vegetariantimes.com/blog/how-to-soak-and-sprout-nuts-seeds-grains-and-beans. If you don't have the time or energy to sprout, simply use nonsprouted beans instead. You can use canned beans or other cooked beans.

Makes 4 servings

2 cups fresh raw corn cut off the cob

1 cup chopped cherry tomatoes

½ cup chopped Mexican Carrots (page 142)

½ cup finely chopped cilantro

1½ cups cooked pinto beans, preferably soaked and sprouted

½ cup chopped olives

3 green onions, chopped, using the white parts and a little of the green stalk

....

Place all of the ingredients in a bowl and mix together thoroughly.

Serve immediately or store in a covered container in the refrigerator for up to 5 days.

CULTURED PICO BEAN DIP

This dish is a variation on the Cultured Peach Pico de Gallo recipe. The addition of corn gives it an extra fresh, summery flavor, and the pinto beans add some filling protein.

A note before you begin: I recommend sprouted beans in this recipe because sprouting ups the nutritional value a great deal. If you'd like to learn how to sprout, visit www .vegetariantimes.com/blog/how-to-soak-and-sprout-nuts-seeds-grains-and-beans. If you don't have the time or energy to sprout, simply use nonsprouted beans instead. You can use canned beans or other cooked beans.

Makes 4 servings

1 cup Cultured Peach Pico de Gallo (page 94)

2 cups fresh raw corn cut off the cob

1½ cups cooked pinto beans, preferably soaked and sprouted

Mix all ingredients together in a bowl and serve immediately or store in a covered container in the refrigerator for up to 5 days.

SCARY-DELICIOUS SEAWEED DIP

Everybody should add some kind of seaweed to their diet. It is one of the healthiest foods on the planet because it's loaded with vitamins, minerals, antioxidants, and iodine, which we all need for a healthy thyroid. This recipe combines seaweed (nori) with cultured veggies. And it was a hit with everybody in my family, even the picky ones. You can serve this with toasted sprouted bread or sprouted chips.

Makes 4 servings

2 sheets nori

1 clove garlic, quartered

2 tablespoons freshly squeezed lemon juice

3 tablespoons olive oil

1 tablespoon toasted sesame oil

½ tablespoon sesame seeds

½ teaspoon Celtic Sea Salt

½ teaspoon freshly ground pepper

2 tablespoons Shelley's Cultured Veggies (page 131)

....

Put the seaweed in a bowl with 1 cup of cold water, and set it aside to rehydrate for 30 minutes.

Drain the seaweed thoroughly and then transfer it to a food processor. Add all remaining ingredients. Pulse until finely chopped.

Serve immediately or store in the refrigerator in a covered bowl for up to 3 days.

WATERMELON PICO DE GALLO

Pico de gallo literally translates as "rooster's beak." Originally it was eaten with the thumb and forefinger, and retrieving and eating the condiment resembled the actions of a pecking rooster. I love this translation as I literally peck at this salad until it is gone. It's crazy good, and just picking out a piece of watermelon leads to a red pepper and on and on—and the next thing I know, I've eaten the whole bowl. You can serve this with sprouted chips—or go nuts and use it on top of grilled chicken or fish.

Makes 12 servings

½ small seedless watermelon, diced

½ red onion, diced

3 cups diced Cultured Red and Yellow Peppers (page 148)

2 jalapeños, seeded and finely diced

1 bunch cilantro, chopped

Juice of 2 limes

½ teaspoon Celtic Sea Salt

Combine all the ingredients in a large bowl and toss to mix.

Serve immediately or store in the refrigerator in an airtight container for up to 1 week.

CHAPTER 9

Main Courses

BUTTERNUT SQUASH AND KEFIR SOUP

When the weather gets cold, I keep a bag of butternut squash in my freezer at all times because I love this soup. It is beyond comfort food; it's heavenly. And leeks add a ton of prebiotics to your diet. Leeks are so effective at feeding your bacteria that I try to eat them as often as I can.

Makes 4 servings

2 tablespoons butter

2 to 3 leeks, cut into rounds

3 ¾ cups chopped fresh or frozen butternut squash

2 tablespoons poultry seasoning

2 ½ teaspoons Celtic Sea Salt

4 cups chicken broth

¾ cup full-fat coconut milk

½ cup Kefir Cheese (page 57)

1 teaspoon black pepper

....

Melt the butter in a pan over medium heat; then add the leeks and sauté until soft.

Add the butternut squash, poultry seasoning, and salt to the pan. Cover with chicken broth and bring the mixture to a boil.

Reduce the heat and simmer until the squash is soft. If using frozen squash, this will take only 5 minutes; fresh squash will take up to 20 minutes.

Remove the mixture from the heat, add the coconut milk, and puree until smooth and creamy, using an immersion hand blender (or a standard blender).

Set the soup aside to cool. When the thermometer reads 100°F or below, ladle into bowls and top each serving with a spoonful of kefir cheese and some black pepper. Adding the cheese while the soup is too hot will kill the probiotics.

CULTURED AVOCADO BOAT

Did you know you could actually live on avocados alone if you wanted to? They have all the nutrition you need. I had no idea of this until I started to look into them. I was craving them all the time, and at first I thought it was because they are high in magnesium. But I think my body was just calling out for more vitamins and minerals in general. This is one of the dishes I came up with when I was in full craving mode. It makes a wonderful lunch because of all the healthy fats and protein—and it has its own bowl!

Makes 2 servings

1 avocado

1 hard-boiled egg, chopped into bite-size pieces

1 tablespoon Shelley's Cultured Veggies (page 131)

2 tablespoons chopped cilantro

1 tablespoon Kefir Cheese (page 57)

½ teaspoon coriander

⅛ teaspoon Celtic Sea Salt

⅛ teaspoon pepper

¼ lime

....

Cut the avocado in half, remove the pit, and scoop out the flesh, making sure to leave the shells intact. Place the avocado flesh in a small bowl.

Add the hard-boiled egg to the avocado.

Add the cultured veggies, cilantro, kefir cheese, coriander, salt, and pepper to the bowl and mix thoroughly.

Scoop the mixture back into the avocado shells and squeeze the lime on top.

COCONUT CURRY STIR-FRY

This is one of my favorite stir-fry dishes. The creamy coconut-milk-and-green-curry topped stir-fry kraut gives you a fantastic meal. You can add cooked chicken or shrimp or just eat it the way it is.

Makes 4 servings

3 cups chopped broccoli

1 cup thinly sliced carrots

2 tablespoons coconut oil

1 small onion, thinly sliced

1 small red bell pepper, seeded and chopped

1 cup full-fat canned coconut milk

1 to 2 tablespoons green curry paste*

2 cups cooked rice

½ cup Stir-Fry Kraut (page 125)

. . . .

Blanch the broccoli and carrots by dunking them in boiling water until tender-crisp, about 1 to 1 ½ minutes. Drain the vegetables and then rinse under cold water to stop the cooking. Drain the vegetables again and set them aside.

Heat the oil in a wok or wide skillet over high heat until hot. Then add the onion and bell pepper. Stir-fry until tender-crisp, about 3 to 4 minutes.

Add the blanched vegetables and toss to mix.

Put the coconut milk and the green curry paste in a blender and mix until smooth.

Add the coconut-curry mixture to the vegetables in the pan and stir to coat.

Pour the mixture over the cooked rice and top with a spoonful of Stir-Fry Kraut.

*Green curry paste can be found in the Asian section of most grocery stores.

PROBIOTIC SWEET POTATO SLIDER

One of my favorite websites is Fit Men Cook, maintained by Kevin Curry. This recipe was inspired by Kevin's Sweet Potato Sliders. I added some probiotic goodness, and what I created is one of my favorite quick meals. Sweet potatoes are so comforting, and these are just fun to eat.

Makes 4 servings

4 wooden skewers

Eight ½-inch-thick slices sweet potato

½ cup fresh spinach leaves

4 thin slices tomato

4 thin slices turkey

2 slices Swiss cheese, cut in half

½ cup Orangeade Kraut (page 137)

¼ cup Billion Bioticland Dressing (page 188)

Preheat the oven to 350°F.

Submerge the wooden skewers in water to soak for at least 1 minute.

Place one piece of the sweet potato on a baking pan. On top of the sweet potato, layer a few spinach leaves, a slice of the tomato, a slice of the turkey, and piece of the Swiss cheese. Top this with another slice of the sweet potato. Push a skewer through the center of the stack, securing all the layers.

Repeat with the remaining ingredients. Cover the pan with aluminum foil. It's okay if the skewers poke through the foil.

Bake until the potatoes are tender, about 25 to 30 minutes. Remove from the oven and cool for 5 minutes or until it feels warm but not hot to the touch.

Remove the skewers, add a spoonful of kraut to the center of each sandwich, and a spoonful of dressing, and then serve immediately.

CULTURED BAKED POTATO

Most of my recipes are super easy because I'm too busy to make complicated meals. Most of us don't have the time, and truth be told, if it's too much work, we won't make and eat foods that are so good for us. While it takes about an hour for the potato in this recipe to bake, you can easily do other things in the meantime. Once the potato is done, prepping the rest of this is lickety-split fast. You don't even have to measure!

Makes 1 serving

1 large russet potato or sweet potato

1 heaping spoonful Lemon Kraut (page 124)

1 large spoonful Kefir Cheese (pages 57)

Black pepper and Celtic Sea Salt to taste

Preheat the oven to 350°F.

Wash the potato thoroughly and use a fork to pierce it eight to ten times. Then place the potato directly on a baking rack in the oven. Bake until you can easily push a fork into the potato, about an hour.

After the potato is baked, split it open lengthwise and let it cool slightly, about 5 minutes. Then top with kraut, kefir cheese, and pepper and salt.

Serve immediately and enjoy.

CRANBERRY WALNUT CHICKPEA SALAD SANDWICH

Some of my favorite food memories are of my teenagers coming in from a day of work, grabbing my leftover chicken salad from the fridge, and telling me about their day. For this recipe I substituted chickpeas for chicken and the results were delicious. Here, I tell you to make a sandwich, but you can put this on a bed of greens for a great salad, too.

A note before you begin: I recommend sprouted beans in this recipe because sprouting ups the nutritional value a great deal. If you'd like to learn how to sprout, visit www .vegetariantimes.com/blog/how-to-soak-and-sprout-nuts-seeds-grains-and-beans. If you don't have the time or energy to sprout, simply use nonsprouted beans instead. You can use canned beans or other cooked beans.

Makes 6 servings

4 tablespoons Basic Kefir (page 51)

1 teaspoon Dijon mustard

1 tablespoon honey or 1 package stevia powder

3 cups cooked garbanzo beans (chickpeas), preferably soaked and sprouted

½ cup diced Fermented Celery with Apples (page 128)

½ cup chopped red grapes

½ cup organic dried cranberries, raisins, or chopped dates

½ cup roughly chopped walnuts or pecans

½ cup thinly sliced green onions

Celtic Sea Salt and freshly ground pepper to taste

6 slices sprouted or sourdough bread (optional)

....

Mix together the kefir, mustard, and honey in a small bowl. Set aside.

Lightly mash the garbanzo beans and celery in a medium bowl with a fork or potato masher. Stir in the grapes, cranberries, nuts, and green onions, and season with salt and pepper.

Pour the kefir mixture into the garbanzo bean mixture and stir until well combined.

Divide the combined mixture among the bread slices and enjoy!

CULTURED TOMATO SOUP

For a few weeks in the springtime my diet consists of mostly raw and cultured foods. I have found that this helps me greatly during allergy season. Although I don't experience many symptoms of hay fever anymore, I find that if I stick to this diet, I fly through the season and feel fantastic! This is one of the soups I love during this time. It fills me up—and I have always thought soup is comfort food.

Makes 1 serving

½ cup Cultured Italian Tomatoes (page 136)

½ cup fresh cherry tomatoes

¼ cup cashews, soaked overnight in water and drained

2 tablespoons Kefir Cheese (page 57)

Add all the ingredients to your blender.

Blend on high for about 90 seconds or until the mixture is smooth. If you have a high-speed blender, this will not only blend the soup but also warm it. If you do not have a high-speed blender, warm the soup over low heat on the stove until a thermometer reads 100°F. Any warmer than this and the probiotics will die.

Pour into a bowl and serve immediately.

RON'S OPEN-FACED CULTURED SANDWICH

I used to make Cultured Italian Tomatoes mostly in the summer so I could use fresh tomatoes. Then my husband, Ron, came up with this combination, which he loves, so now I have to make them all year round!

Makes 1 serving

1 slice sourdough bread

½ cup Kefir Cheese (page 57)

½ cup chopped Cultured Italian Tomatoes (page 136)

2 fresh basil leaves

½ teaspoon Celtic Sea Salt

1 tablespoon olive oil

Toast the sourdough bread and spread the kefir cheese on top.

Top with the tomatoes and basil, sprinkle with the salt, and drizzle the olive oil on top.

TORTILLA SOUP

The first time I had this soup (a noncultured version of it) was at a store demonstration for a high-speed Blendtec blender. I was so impressed that I plunked down several hundred dollars right then and there for my own, and I've never looked back. This is the best appliance I own. It can blend all kinds of fruits and veggies no matter how dense or bulky they are. I honestly can't imagine life without it now. That said, you don't need a high-speed blender to make this recipe.

Makes 2 servings

2 Roma tomatoes

½ cup Mexican Carrots (page 142)

⅓ cup chopped red pepper

½ avocado

2 tablespoons chopped onion

½ cup pepper jack cheese

2 sprigs cilantro

¾ teaspoon Celtic Sea Salt

¼ cup Kefir Cheese (page 57)

1 teaspoon chili powder

¾ teaspoon garlic powder

½ cup tortilla chips

....

Add all of the ingredients (except the tortilla chips) plus two cups of warm water to the blender. Blend on high for about 90 seconds or until the mixture is smooth.

Add the tortilla chips and pulse 2 or 3 times.

If you have a high-speed blender, the blending will not only blend the soup but also warm it. If you do not have a high-speed blender, warm the soup over low heat on the stove until a thermometer reads 100°F. Any warmer than this and the probiotics will die. Pour into bowls and serve.

CULTURED VEGGIE BIG BOWL

This beautiful array of veggies has such an interesting blend of tastes and textures that it will suit anyone. Sweet and sour, soft and crunchy—I love the combinations! And if you plate this with each ingredient separate, it makes a really pretty presentation.

Makes 1 serving

1 sweet potato

½ avocado

½ cup mixed greens or kale

¼ cup garbanzo beans (chickpeas)

¼ cup Carrots with Orange Peel (page 135)

2 tablespoons Lemon Kefir Labneh (page 183)

3 tablespoons Kefir Ranch Dressing (page 185)

2 tablespoons pumpkin seeds or chopped pecans

....

Preheat the oven to 400°F.

Wash the sweet potato thoroughly and pierce it eight to ten times with a fork. Then place it directly on a baking rack in the oven and bake until you can easily push a fork into it, about 45 minutes.

Let the sweet potato cool. Meanwhile, chop the avocado and greens into bite-size pieces. When the sweet potato is cool enough to handle, cut it into bite-size pieces.

Place the sweet potato, avocado, greens, chickpeas, and carrots around the outside of a large bowl, keeping each vegetable separate and leaving space in the center.

Add the labneh to the center and drizzle the ranch dressing over the entire dish. Sprinkle with pumpkin seeds and serve.

VEGGIE DELIGHT

I could eat this super-yummy sandwich every day of my life and never tire of it. My Billion Bioticland Dressing makes it something special. It tastes like Thousand Island dressing but has billions of probiotics in it.

Makes 1 serving

2 tablespoons Billion Bioticland Dressing (page 188)

2 slices sprouted or sourdough bread

2 slices Swiss cheese

½ avocado, peeled and sliced into long pieces

1 large portobello mushroom, sliced into several pieces

¼ cup Orangeade Kraut, well drained (page 137)

1 tablespoon butter

....

Spread the dressing on the bread.

Place one slice of Swiss cheese on one slice of the bread.

Add the avocado, mushroom, and kraut.

Top with the other piece of cheese and slice of bread.

Grill the sandwich on a panini grill or skillet, cooking it just until the cheese melts. This will ensure that it does not reach a temperature that will kill the probiotics.

Serve immediately.

CASHEW KEFIR ITALIAN CHEESECAKE

I served savory cheesecake at Christmas, and my daughter Maci is now obsessed with it. Its flavor is quite unique, and it stimulates all your taste buds—sweet, salty, and sour. It's also a pretty dish that you can make to impress your friends. In my house, we eat this as a main course and as a side. Either way, it's delicious!

Makes 6 servings

For the crust

1 cup walnuts

1 cup raisins

1 tablespoon coconut oil

For the filling

2 cups raw cashews, soaked overnight in water and drained

½ cup Basic Kefir (page 51)

½ teaspoon Celtic Sea Salt

½ cup fresh basil

1 teaspoon lemon juice

For the topping

½ cup Cultured Italian Tomatoes (page 136)

¼ cup balsamic vinegar

1 cup basil, chopped

To make the crust, place the walnuts and raisins in a food processor and pulse until the mixture resembles small crumbs.

Add the coconut oil and pulse again until the mixture sticks together.

Press this mixture into a 7-inch springform pan.

For the filling, add the cashews to a food processor and pulse until nuts are finely ground. Add the kefir, salt, basil, and lemon juice and pulse again until the mixture is smooth.

Place the cashew mixture on top of the crust. Cover the pan with plastic wrap and place it in the refrigerator for at least 4 hours.

Remove the cashew cheesecake from the fridge. Top with the Cultured Italian Tomatoes, drizzle with balsamic vinegar, and sprinkle with chopped basil.

Serve immediately.

MIRACLE KRAUT MELT

I went to a wonderful restaurant in Denver and had a sandwich that was the inspiration for this recipe. Melted cheese and kraut is a genius combination! But remember, you have to grill this open-faced so you can add the kraut after grilling and not kill the probiotics. I'm so thankful I went to that restaurant. Not only did they have this sandwich, but they also had kombucha on tap and kimchi stew! It's wonderful to see cultured foods popping up on menus around the country. People are starting to fall in love with fermentation—as they rightfully should!

Makes 1 serving

1 tablespoon butter

2 slices sourdough or sprouted bread

2 slices cheddar cheese or 4 ounces goat cheese or Brie

⅓ cup Thank-You Kraut (page 126)

....

Butter one side of each slice of bread, taking care to spread the butter to the very edges.

Heat a skillet over medium-low heat, then place the slices of bread in the skillet, buttered side down.

Add half the cheese to each slice of bread.

When the cheese is melted and the bread is lightly browned, remove both slices from pan and let them cool for a minute of two.

Layer kraut on one slice, then place the other slice on top and press them together.

Cut the sandwich in half and serve immediately.

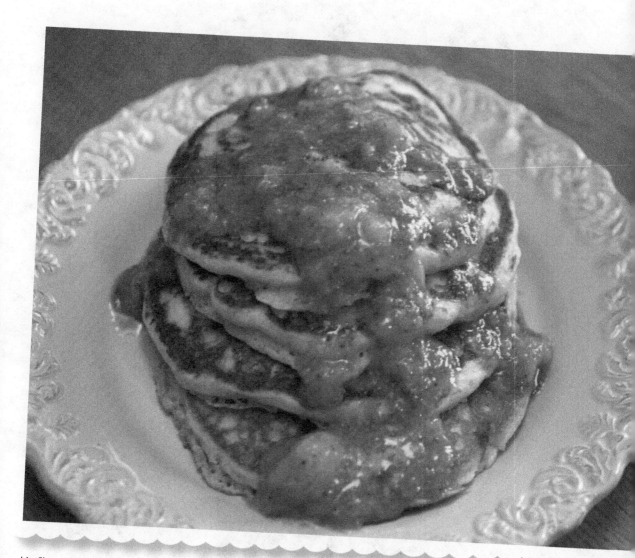

Kefir Pancakes, page 83.

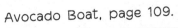

Avocado Boat, page 109.

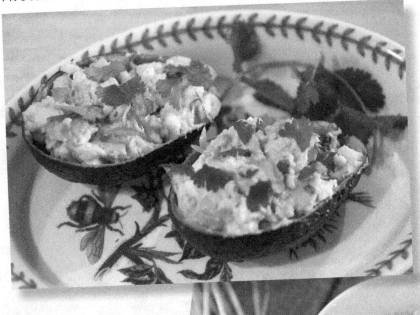

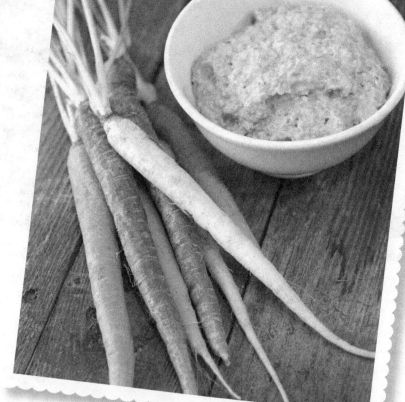

Earth and Sunshine Dip, page 100.

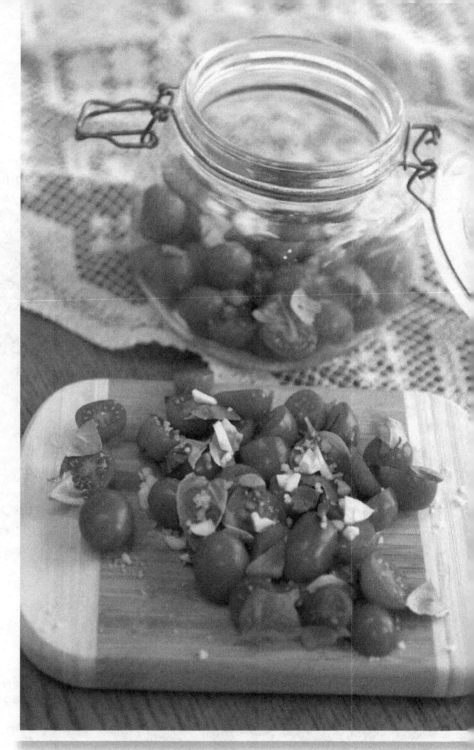

Cultured Itatlian Tomatoes, page 136.

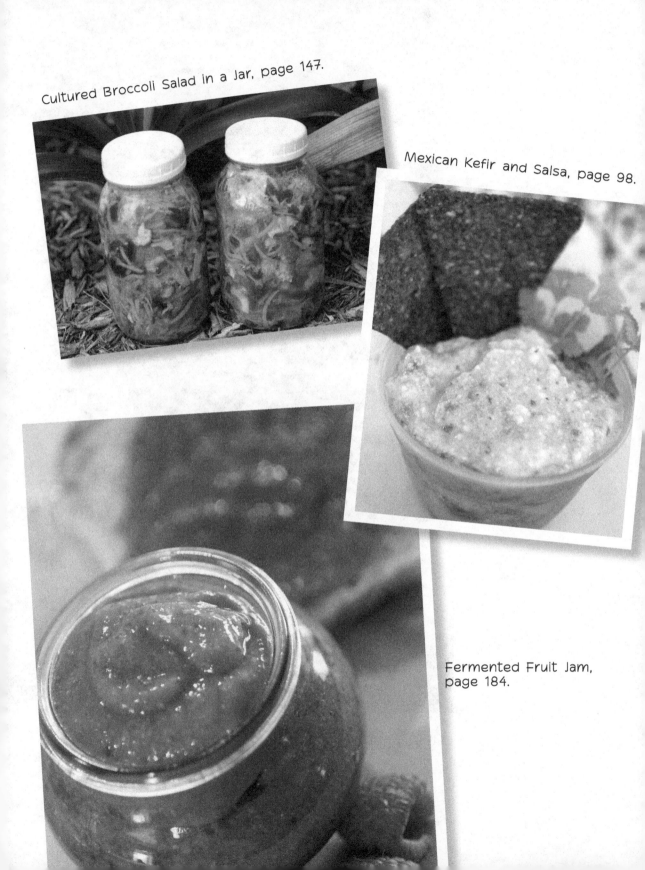

Cultured Broccoli Salad in a Jar, page 147.

Mexican Kefir and Salsa, page 98.

Fermented Fruit Jam, page 184.

Cultured Veggie Big Bowl, page 117.

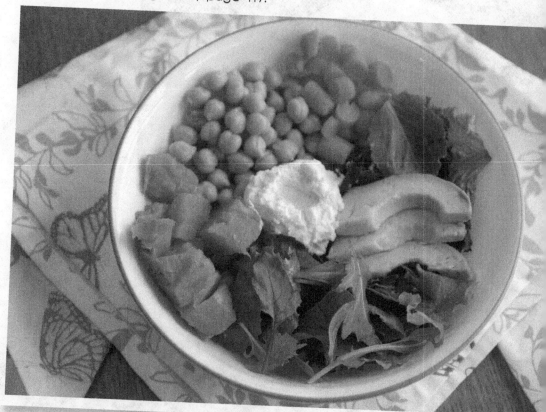

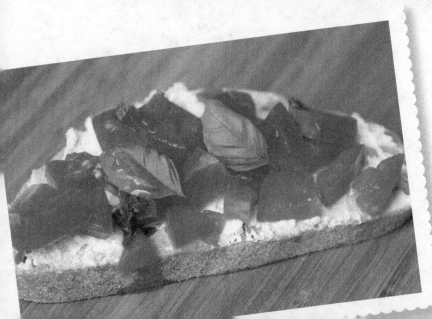

Ron's Open Face
Cultured Sandwich,
page 115.

Kefir Orange Cups, page 95.

Veggies Love Kefir Cheese, page 99.

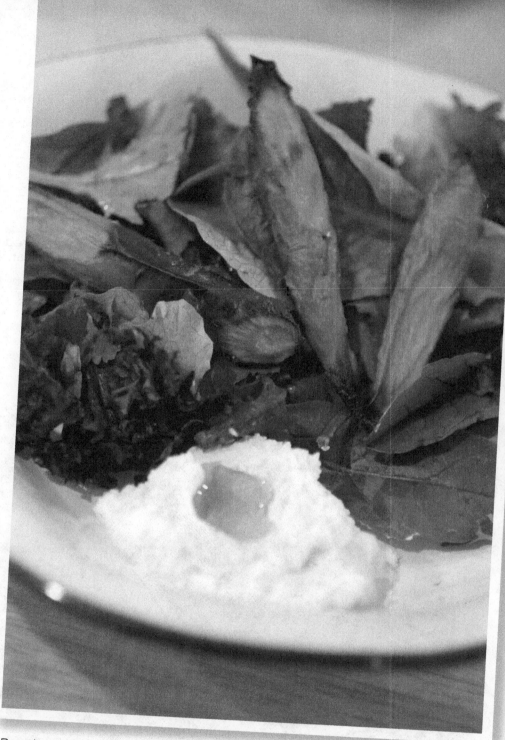

Roasted Carrot Kefir Salad, page 123.

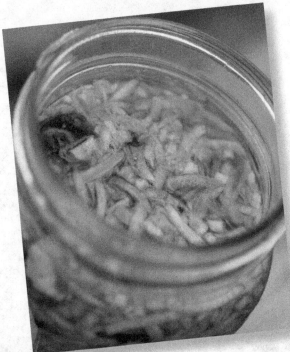

Cultured Carrot Cake
in a Jar, page 149.

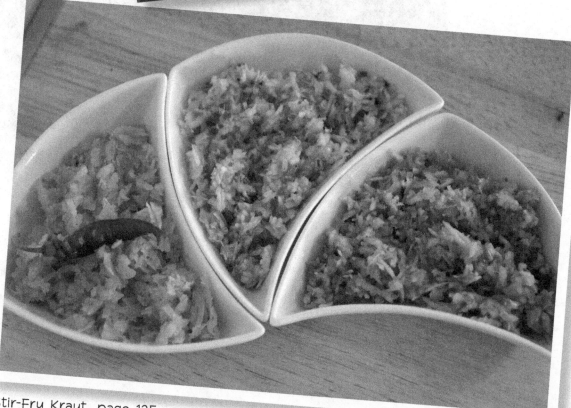

Stir-Fry Kraut, page 125;
Buffalo Kraut, page 129;
Thank-You Kraut, page 126.

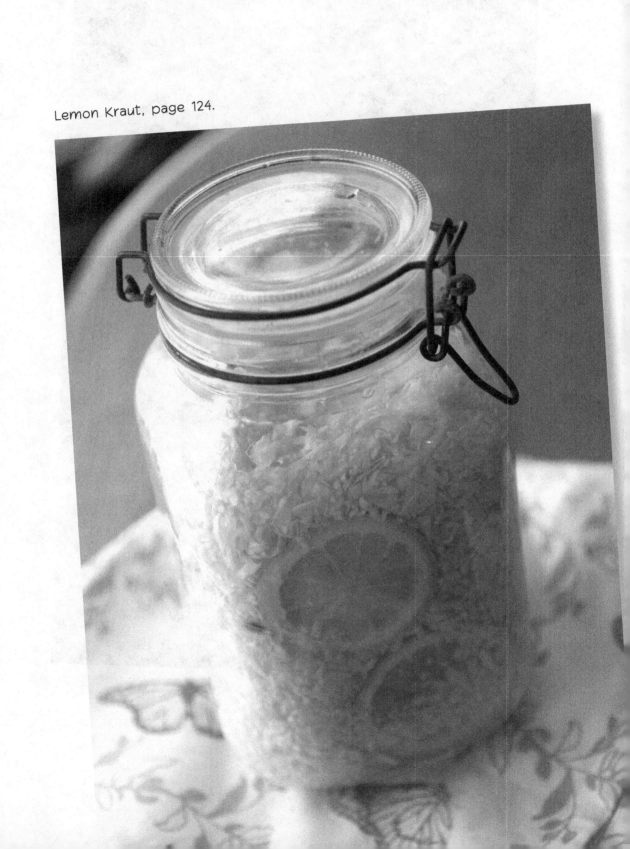

Lemon Kraut, page 124.

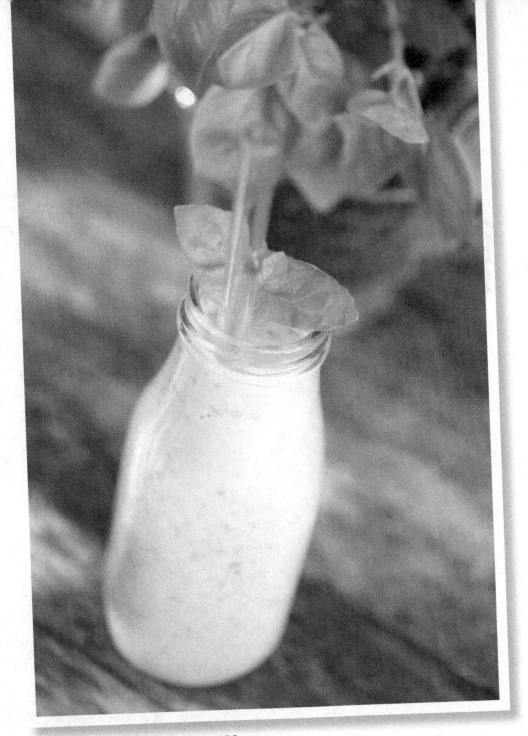

Sun-Fresh Smoothie, page 82.

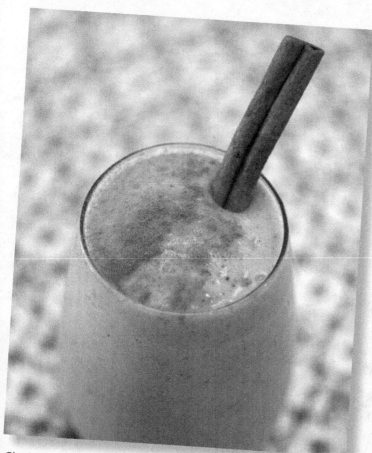

Chai Kefir Smoothie, page 71.

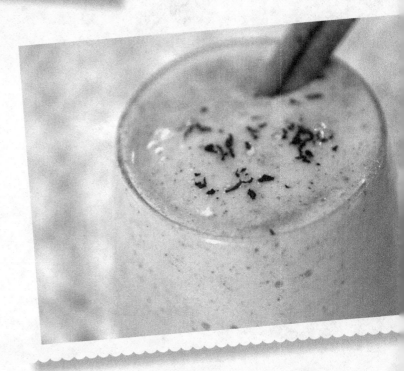

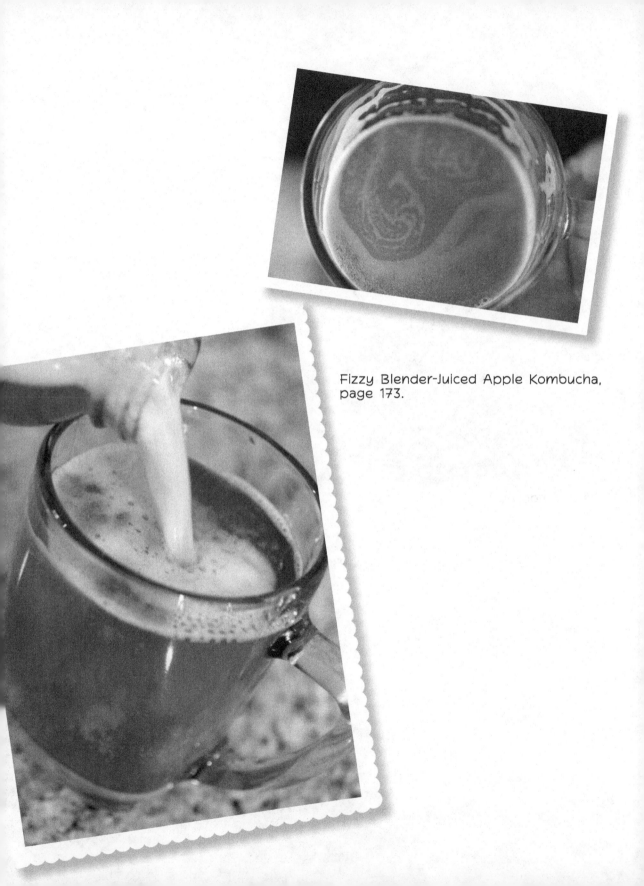

Fizzy Blender-Juiced Apple Kombucha,
page 173.

Chocolate Kefir Coconut Pudding, page 162.

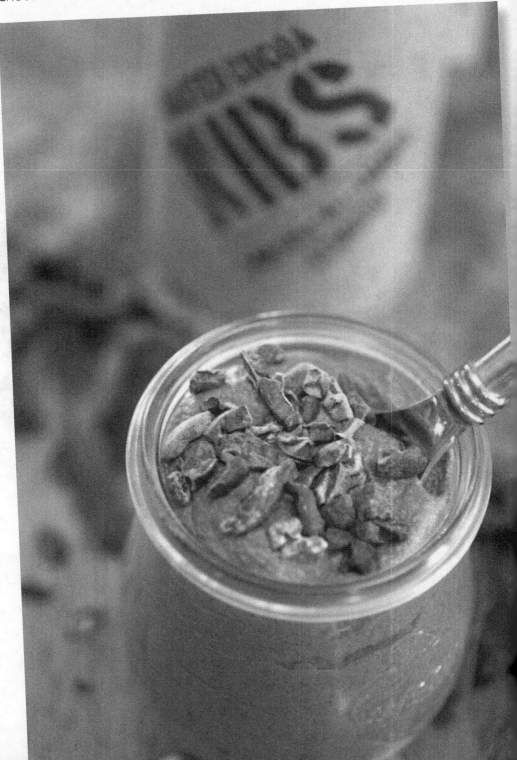

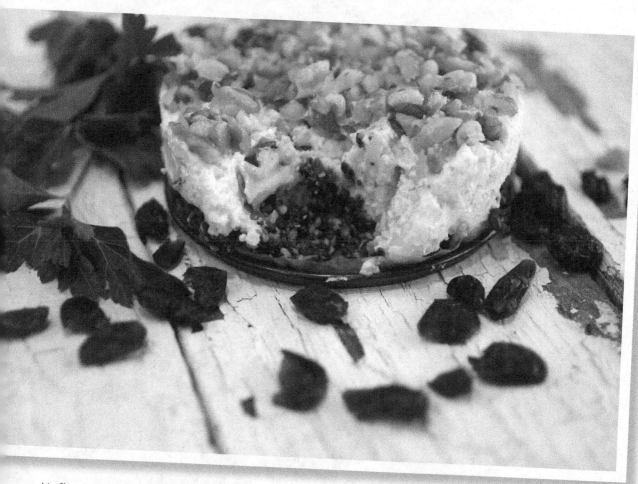

Kefir Cheese and Veggie Torte, page 89.

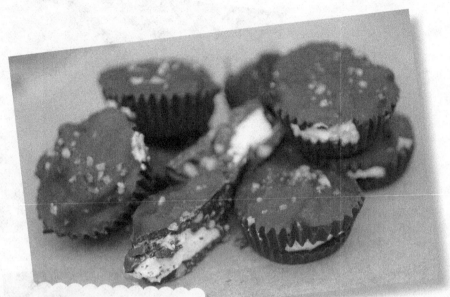

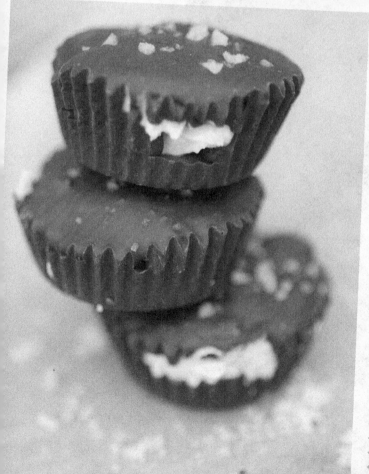

Chocolate Kefir Candy,
page 153.

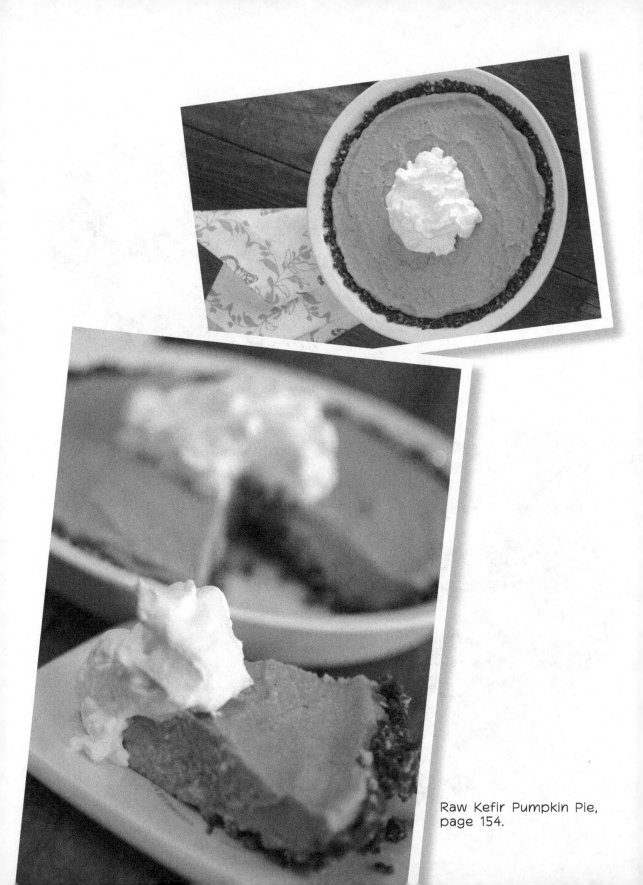

Raw Kefir Pumpkin Pie,
page 154.

Side Dishes and Salads

KEFIR CAESAR SALAD

Anchovies are an ingredient that makes Caesar salad incredible. They are also super healthy because they're high in omega-3s. But I say they're a secret ingredient here because you can't really taste them in this salad. Case in point: My husband asked me one day why I wanted him to buy anchovies at the store. "After all," he said, "I would never eat anchovies." To which I replied, "You eat them all the time; you just don't know it!"

Makes 4 servings

For the salad

1 large head romaine lettuce
⅛ cup grated, fresh Parmigiano-Reggiano cheese

For the Kefir Caesar Dressing

⅓ cup Basic Kefir (page 51)
2 anchovy fillets, mashed
1 clove garlic, minced
2 tablespoons fresh lemon juice
2 teaspoons Worcestershire sauce
2 tablespoons extra-virgin olive oil

⅛ cup grated, fresh Parmigiano-Reggiano cheese

Celtic Sea Salt and pepper to taste

....

Tear the lettuce into bite-size pieces and put them in a large bowl.

To make the dressing, mix together the kefir, anchovy fillets, garlic, lemon juice, and Worcestershire sauce, using a wire whisk. Then whisk in the olive oil, ⅛ cup cheese, and salt and pepper.

Toss the salad with the dressing, top with the remaining ⅛ cup cheese, and serve immediately.

ROASTED CARROT KEFIR SALAD

Generally I don't think of salad as a comfort food, but this one might actually qualify. The caramelized carrots with a side of Lemon Kefir Labneh, and a cultured dressing make it not only delicious but also satisfyingly filling. It can be eye-catching, too, if you make it with multicolored rainbow carrots. When I did this, it was so beautiful I almost didn't want to eat it.

Makes 2 servings

½ pound carrots

3 tablespoons olive oil + more for garnish

1 teaspoon Celtic Sea Salt

½ teaspoon black pepper

4 cups mixed greens

⅓ cup Kefir Caesar Dressing (page 121)

½ cup Lemon Kefir Labneh (page 183)

....

Preheat the oven to 400°F.

Wash the carrots and cut them diagonally into 1½-inch slices.

Place the carrots in a bowl and toss them with the olive oil, salt, and pepper.

Place the carrots on a baking sheet in one layer and roast for 20 minutes.

Place the mixed greens on two plates and top with the roasted carrots. Drizzle the dressing over the salad and top with a dollop of the kefir labneh. Drizzle a little olive oil on top and serve.

LEMON KRAUT

Lemons are superfoods: they are a digestive aid and a liver cleanser, and they contain many nutritional substances such as citric acid, calcium, magnesium, vitamin C, bioflavonoids, and pectin. All this goodness promotes immunity and fights infections. And the peels act as a prebiotic!

Makes 2 quarts; 32 ¼-cup servings

¼ teaspoon Cutting Edge Starter Culture plus ½ cup water, or ¼ cup Kefir Whey (page 57)

1 small cabbage (about 1 pound)

1 apple, unpeeled and cored

1 tablespoon Celtic Sea Salt

1 lemon, sliced

If using the starter culture, stir together the culture and water. Let the mixture sit while you prepare the other ingredients—around 10 minutes.

Remove and discard the outer leaves of the cabbage. Finely shred the cabbage and apple, using a food processor or a hand shredder. Place the mixture in a bowl.

Add the salt to the cabbage and apple and set the mixture aside.

Line the inside of the jar with lemon slices, then pack the cabbage and apple into the middle of the jar.

Add the starter culture or the whey and fill the jar with filtered water, leaving 2 to 3 inches of headspace to let the cabbage mixture bubble and expand as it ferments.

Seal the container and let it sit on your kitchen counter, out of direct sunlight, for 6 days.

Check the kraut every day to make sure it is fully submerged. If it has risen above the water, simply push it down so it is fully covered again. If white spots of yeast have formed on any unsubmerged pieces, do not worry. Remember, this isn't harmful. Just scoop out the yeast and the kraut it's on and push the rest back under the water. (See FAQs on page 69 for more information.)

When the kraut is done fermenting, place it in the refrigerator.

Storage note: This kraut can be kept in an airtight jar in the refrigerator for up to 9 months.

STIR-FRY KRAUT

This recipe is a great garnish for any stir-fry dish. It uses a spicy Asian sauce called Sriracha, which is made from hot peppers, garlic, and other seasonings. You can find this in most grocery stores nowadays.

Makes 2 quarts; 32 ¼-cup servings

¼ teaspoon Cutting Edge Starter Culture plus ½ cup water, or ¼ cup Kefir Whey (page 57)

¼ head small cabbage

¼ onion

2 red kung pao peppers

2 tablespoons soy sauce

1 tablespoon sesame oil

1 teaspoon Sriracha

1 teaspoon red pepper flakes

If using the starter culture, stir together the culture and water. Let the mixture sit while you prepare the other ingredients—around 10 minutes.

Remove and discard the outer leaves of the cabbage. Finely shred the cabbage, onion, and hot peppers (you can seed them first if you like less spice) using a food processor or a hand shredder.

Pack the cabbage mixture into a jar.

Add the soy sauce, sesame oil, Sriracha, and red pepper flakes.

Add the starter culture or the whey and fill the jar with filtered water, leaving 2 to 3 inches of headspace to let the cabbage mixture bubble and expand as it ferments.

Seal the container and let it sit on your kitchen counter, out of direct sunlight, for 6 days.

Check the kraut every day to make sure it is fully submerged. If it has risen above the water, simply push it down so it is fully covered again. If white spots of yeast have formed on any unsubmerged kraut, do not worry. Remember, this isn't harmful. Just scoop out the yeast and kraut it's on and push the rest back under the water. (See FAQs on page 69 for more information.)

When the kraut is done fermenting, place it in the refrigerator.

Storage note: This kraut can be kept in an airtight jar in the refrigerator for up to 9 months.

THANK-YOU KRAUT

We named this Thank-You Kraut because it is perfect for Thanksgiving. It's loaded with cranberries and cranberry juice, which give it quite a unique flavor. You can serve it as a side dish or with crackers or a veggie platter. Or, if you're like me, you can pile it on top of leftover turkey and sourdough to make a delicious probiotic sandwich. You'll be thankful you did.

Makes 2 quarts; 32 ¼-cup servings

¼ teaspoon Cutting Edge Starter Culture plus ½ cup water, or ¼ cup Kefir Whey (page 57)

½ small head cabbage

1½ teaspoons Celtic Sea Salt

½ cup cranberries

1 cup cranberry juice

....

If using the starter culture, stir together the culture and water. Let the mixture sit while you prepare the other ingredients—around 10 minutes.

Remove and discard the outer leaves of the cabbage. Finely shred or chop the cabbage into bite-sized pieces, using a food processor or a hand shredder. Place the shredded cabbage in a large bowl.

Mix in the salt, cranberries, and cranberry juice and pack the mixture into a jar.

Add the starter culture or the whey and fill the jar with filtered water, leaving 2 to 3 inches of headspace to let the cabbage mixture bubble and expand as it ferments.

Seal the container and let it sit on your kitchen counter, out of direct sunlight, for 6 days.

Check the kraut every day to make sure it is fully submerged. If it has risen above the water, simply push it down so it is fully covered again. If white spots of yeast have formed on any unsubmerged kraut, do not worry. Remember, this isn't harmful. Just scoop out the yeast and kraut it's on and push the rest back under the water. (See FAQs on page 69 for more information.)

When the kraut is done fermenting, place it in the refrigerator.

Storage note: This kraut can be kept in an airtight jar in the refrigerator for up to 9 months.

FLU-PREVENTION CULTURED VEGETABLES

This recipe was in my last book, but it's so powerful that I wanted to include it again. Since the time I published that book, I learned just why it is so good at fighting the flu: prebiotics! When I first made this, I knew nothing about prebiotics; I just knew that this recipe provided spectacular healing results. And remember: the juice is just as powerful as the vegetables. Just a spoonful can start you toward feeling better—or, better yet, prevent you from getting sick in the first place.

Makes 2 quarts; 32 ¼-cup servings

¼ teaspoon Cutting Edge Starter Culture plus ½ cup water, or ¼ cup Kefir Whey (page 57)
½ small head cabbage
1 medium jicama, peeled
3 handfuls fresh spinach
1 medium apple, cored
1 small white onion
1 clove garlic
1½ teaspoons Celtic Sea Salt
Zest and juice of 1 large orange

If using the starter culture, stir together the culture and water. Let the mixture sit while you prepare the other ingredients—around 10 minutes.

Remove and discard the outer leaves of the cabbage. Shred or chop the cabbage, jicama, spinach, apple, onion, and garlic. Place them in a large bowl and sprinkle with the salt.

Firmly pack the vegetable mixture into two 1-quart glass or ceramic containers that can be securely sealed.

Add half the orange zest and juice and half the culture or kefir whey to each jar. Then fill the containers with filtered water, leaving 2 inches of headspace to let the vegetables bubble and expand as they ferment.

Seal the containers and let them sit on your kitchen counter, out of direct sunlight, for 6 days.

Check the vegetables every day to make sure they are fully submerged. If they have risen above the water, simply push them down so they are fully covered again. If any white spots of yeast have formed on any unsubmerged vegetables, do not worry. Remember, this isn't harmful. Just scoop out the yeast and vegetables it's on and push the rest back under the water. (See FAQs on page 69 for more information.)

When the veggies are done fermenting, place them in the refrigerator.

Storage note: These veggies can be stored in an airtight container in the refrigerator for up to 9 months.

FERMENTED CELERY WITH APPLES

A lot of people think of celery as boring, but it actually has quite a few health benefits, such as being extremely high in vitamin K. It has also been very helpful in lowering blood pressure in people with hypertension. In this recipe, you lose celery's boringness by mixing it with ginger and apple. The flavors blend together so well that you may never think poorly of celery again!

Makes 2 quarts; 32 ¼-cup servings

¼ teaspoon Cutting Edge Starter Culture plus ½ cup water, or ¼ cup Kefir Whey (page 57)

1 large bunch celery

1 apple

1-inch piece ginger

....

If using the starter culture, stir together the culture and water. Let the mixture sit while you prepare the other ingredients—around 10 minutes.

Trim the celery, cut it into bite-size pieces, and put the pieces in a jar.

Core the apple and chop it into small pieces, and add it to the jar. Then add the whole piece of ginger.

Add the culture and fill the container with filtered water, leaving 2 inches of headspace to let the contents bubble and expand as they ferment.

Seal the container and let it sit on your kitchen counter, out of direct sunlight, for 6 days.

Check the celery every day to make sure it is fully submerged. If it has risen above the water, simply push it down so it is fully covered again. If white spots of yeast have formed on any unsubmerged celery, do not worry. Remember, this isn't harmful. Just scoop out the yeast and celery it's on and push the rest back under the water. (See FAQs on page 69 for more information.)

When the celery is done fermenting, place it in the refrigerator.

Storage note: This celery can be stored in an airtight container in the refrigerator for up to 9 months.

BUFFALO KRAUT

Buffalo wings are all the rage these days. But did you know that the first plate of wings was served in 1964 at a family-owned establishment in Buffalo called the Anchor Bar? The wings were the brainchild of Teressa Bellissimo—she covered some wings with her own special sauce and served them with a side of blue cheese and celery because that's what she had available. Inspired by this, my daughter Maci took the same ingredients (minus the chicken wings) and made a delicious veggie recipe.

Makes 2 quarts; 32 ¼-cup servings

¼ teaspoon Cutting Edge Starter Culture plus ½ cup water, or ¼ cup Kefir Whey (page 57)

½ large head cabbage

2 stalks celery

½ cup buffalo sauce

½ tablespoon onion powder

1 tablespoon chopped chives

1 tablespoon Celtic Sea Salt

Blue cheese crumbles

....

If using the starter culture, stir together the culture and water. Let the mixture sit while you prepare the other ingredients—around 10 minutes.

Remove and discard the outer leaves of the cabbage. Shred the cabbage and place it in a bowl. Then chop the celery into small pieces and mix it with the cabbage.

Mix in the buffalo sauce, onion powder, and chives until well combined. Put the mixture in a jar.

Add the culture and fill the container with filtered water, leaving 2 inches of headspace to let the vegetables bubble and expand as they ferment.

Seal the container and let it sit on your kitchen counter, out of direct sunlight, for 6 days.

Check the kraut every day to make sure it is fully submerged. If it has risen above the water, simply push it down so it is fully covered again. If white spots of yeast have formed on any unsubmerged kraut, do not worry. Remember, this isn't harmful. Just scoop out the yeast and kraut it's on and push the rest back under the water. (See FAQs on page 69 for more information.)

When the kraut is done fermenting, place it in the refrigerator.

Serve with a small amount of blue cheese crumbles.

Storage note: These veggies can be stored in an airtight container in the refrigerator for up to 9 months.

KEFIR ALMOND BREAD

This is my yummy alternative to conventional bread, and it's great for anybody who wants an easy, gluten-free recipe. I love having a couple of slices topped with Fermented Fruit Jam (page 184) in the morning. That and a pot of my favorite tea are a great way to start the day!

Makes 1 loaf; 8 servings

3 ½ cups almond flour

¼ cup butter, melted

3 eggs

1 teaspoon baking soda

¼ teaspoon Celtic Sea Salt

1 cup Basic Kefir (page 51)

2 tablespoons ground flaxseed

Preheat the oven to 350°F.

Mix all the ingredients in a medium-size bowl.

Place the mixture in a greased loaf pan and bake for 45 minutes.

Remove it from the pan and cool it on a wire rack.

SHELLEY'S CULTURED VEGGIES

This is one of the most popular recipes at my house. It is even more wonderful with a scoop of EcoBloom, which enhances the flavor and gives you prebiotics, too. Shelley, who gave me this recipe, is a dear friend and someone who was there to support me when I was writing my very first book. I love all my cultured-food friends, who come up with the best recipes.

Makes 1 gallon; 64 ¼-cup servings

1 packet Cutting Edge Starter Culture plus 1 cup water, or ½ cup Kefir Whey (page 57)

1 large head green cabbage

6 carrots

½ white onion

½ Granny Smith apple

1 cup kale leaves or spinach leaves

2 tablespoons dried parsley or 4 tablespoons chopped fresh parsley

2 tablespoons Bragg Organic Sea Kelp Delight Seasoning, or more to taste

2 teaspoons Celtic Sea Salt, or more to taste

1 clove garlic, minced, or more to taste

....

If using the starter culture, stir together the culture and water. Let the mixture sit while you prepare the other ingredients—around 10 minutes.

Remove and discard the outer leaves from the cabbage. Chop the cabbage, carrots, and onions into small pieces and place them in the work bowl of a food processor.

Core the apple and chop it into small pieces. Add these to the food processor and pulse until grated. Transfer the mixture to a large bowl.

Chop the kale.

Add the kale, parsley, sea kelp seasoning, salt, and garlic to the large bowl and mix the veggies until thoroughly combined.

Pack the mixture into glass or ceramic containers that can be securely sealed. Press the vegetables down into the jar with your hand, a wooden spoon, or a potato masher.

Divide the culture or whey among the containers. Then fill the containers with filtered water, leaving 2 inches of headspace to let the vegetables bubble and expand as they ferment.

Seal the containers and let them sit on your kitchen counter, out of direct sunlight, for 6 days.

Check the vegetables every day to make sure they are fully submerged. If they have risen above the water, simply push them down so they are fully covered again. If white spots of yeast have formed on any unsubmerged vegetables, do not worry. Remember, this isn't harmful. Just scoop out the yeast and vegetables it's on and push the rest back under the water. (See FAQs on page 69 for more information.)

When the veggies are done fermenting, place them in the refrigerator.

Storage note: These veggies can be stored in airtight containers in the refrigerator for up to 9 months.

CURTIDO SALVADORAN KRAUT

Curtido is a fermented cabbage dish popular in Central America. It is served alongside pupusas, which are thick, handmade corn tortillas filled with cheese, beans, and meat. I completely understand why curtido is considered a national delicacy—the sweet-and-sour taste and the flavor of lime in this kraut are exceptional. I think you will love it.

Makes 2 quarts; 32 ¼-cup servings

¼ teaspoon Cutting Edge Starter Culture plus ½ cup water, or ¼ cup Kefir Whey (page 57)

½ head cabbage

1 large carrot

½ onion

¼ cup lime juice

½ teaspoon Celtic Sea Salt

2 tablespoons Sucanat or coconut sugar

1 teaspoon dried oregano (preferably Mexican)

½ to 1 teaspoon red pepper flakes

If using the starter culture, stir together the culture and water. Let the mixture sit while you prepare the other ingredients—around 10 minutes.

Remove and discard the outer leaves of the cabbage. Shred the cabbage and place it in a bowl. Then shred the carrot and onion and mix them with the cabbage.

Add the lime juice, salt, Sucanat, oregano, and red pepper flakes until well combined. Put the mixture in a jar.

Add the culture or kefir whey and fill the container with filtered water, leaving 2 inches of headspace to let the vegetables bubble and expand as they ferment.

Seal the container and let it sit on your kitchen counter, out of direct sunlight, for 6 days.

Check the kraut every day to make sure it is fully submerged. If it has risen above the water, simply push it down so it is fully covered again. If white spots of yeast have formed on any unsubmerged kraut, do not worry. Remember, this isn't harmful. Just scoop out the yeast and kraut it's on and push the rest back under the water. (See FAQs on page 69 for more information.)

When the kraut is done fermenting, place it in the refrigerator.

Storage note: These veggies can be stored in an airtight container in the refrigerator for up to 9 months.

SPICY CULTURED BEETS AND HONEY

This recipe was given to me by my friend Shelley, who also invented Shelley's Cultured Vegetables (page 131). She has a flair for making great cultured-veggie combinations. This one is especially good around the holidays because of its festive red color. I use it like cranberry sauce; sometimes I even add a few tablespoons of dried cranberries for a fun twist.

Makes 1 quart; 16 ¼-cup servings

⅛ teaspoon Cutting Edge Starter Culture plus ¼ cup water, or 2 tablespoons Kefir Whey (page 57)

1 tablespoon raw honey

4 medium beets

1-inch piece ginger

Zest from 1 medium orange

1 teaspoon whole allspice berries

1 teaspoon whole black peppercorns

1 teaspoon whole cloves

2 sticks cinnamon

....

If using the starter culture, stir together the culture and water. Add the honey and mix until it is dissolved. If using whey, mix the whey and honey together. Let the mixture sit while you prepare the other ingredients—around 10 minutes.

Peel the beets and slice them into ⅛-inch rounds.

Peel the ginger and cut it into matchsticks.

Place the beets, ginger, orange zest, and spices in a mixing bowl and stir to combine.

Transfer the veggie mixture to a jar and add the starter culture mixture or the whey. Then fill the jar with filtered water, leaving 2 to 3 inches of headspace to let the beets bubble and expand as they ferment.

Seal the container and let it sit on your kitchen counter, out of direct sunlight, for 3 to 5 days.

Check the beets every day to make sure they are fully submerged. If they have risen above the water, simply push them down so they are fully covered again. If white spots of yeast have formed on any unsubmerged beets, do not worry. Remember, this isn't harmful. Just scoop out the yeast and beets it's on and push the rest back under the water. (See FAQs on page 69 for more information.)

When the beets are done fermenting, place them in the refrigerator.

Storage note: These beets can be kept in an airtight jar in the refrigerator for up to 9 months.

CARROTS WITH ORANGE PEEL

This is my favorite way to make carrots. The sweetness of the carrots with the zing of orange makes a combo that even the pickiest eaters will enjoy. You can leave the carrots whole or you can chop them up. You can even ferment baby carrots if you're making it for your little ones.

Makes 1 quart; 16 ¼-cup servings

⅛ teaspoon Cutting Edge Starter Culture plus ¼ cup water, or 2 tablespoons Kefir Whey (page 57)

4 or 5 carrots

Orange peel, one long strip

1/2 teaspoon Celtic Sea Salt

....

If using the starter culture, stir together the culture and water. Let the mixture sit while you prepare the other ingredients—around 10 minutes.

Trim the carrots, cut them into pieces, and put them in your jar.

Add the orange peel and salt.

Add the starter culture or the whey and fill the jar with filtered water, leaving 2 to 3 inches of headspace to let the carrots bubble and expand as they ferment.

Seal the container and let it sit on your kitchen counter, out of direct sunlight, for 3 days.

Check the carrots every day to make sure they are fully submerged. If they have risen above the water, simply push them down so they are fully covered again. If white spots of yeast have formed on any unsubmerged carrots, do not worry. Remember, this isn't harmful. Just scoop out the yeast and carrots it's on and push the rest back under the water. (See FAQs on page 69 for more information.)

When the carrots are done fermenting, place them in the refrigerator.

Storage note: These carrots can be kept in an airtight jar in the refrigerator for up to 9 months.

CULTURED ITALIAN TOMATOES

I served these at my daughter's wedding shower, and they were gobbled up so fast I couldn't believe it. And everybody was asking for more. That shouldn't have surprised me, because it was summer—just the right time for this dish, which is fabulous and made with tomatoes straight from the vine. This recipe is a great one to start with when you're preparing cultured vegetables for the first time.

Makes 1 quart; 16 ¼-cup servings

⅛ teaspoon Cutting Edge Starter Culture plus ¼ cup water, or 2 tablespoons Kefir Whey (page 57)

1 clove garlic

3 cups halved cherry tomatoes

¼ cup chopped fresh basil

1 teaspoon Celtic Sea Salt

If using the starter culture, stir together the culture and water. Let the mixture sit while you prepare the other ingredients—around 10 minutes.

Mince the garlic; then place the garlic, tomatoes, basil, and salt in a bowl and toss to combine.

Transfer the mixture to your jar and add the starter culture or the whey. Then fill the jar with filtered water, leaving 2 to 3 inches of headspace to let the carrots bubble and expand as they ferment.

Seal the container and let it sit on your kitchen counter, out of direct sunlight, for 2 days.

Check the tomatoes every day to make sure they are fully submerged. If they have risen above the water, simply push them down so they are fully covered again. If white spots of yeast have formed on any unsubmerged tomatoes, do not worry. Remember, this isn't harmful. Just scoop out the yeast and tomatoes it's on and push the rest back under the water. (See FAQs on page 69 for more information.)

When the tomatoes are done fermenting, place them in the refrigerator.

Storage note: These tomatoes can be kept in an airtight jar in the refrigerator for up to 3 months.

ORANGEADE KRAUT

This is my most popular cultured veggie recipe and the one I teach people to make at my classes. It's visually beautiful, and also it's one of the most delicious krauts you'll ever have. Oranges, apples, and cabbage give it a sweet-and-sour taste that is perfect as a side dish with a meal. For the last three years I have had a jar of this in my fridge at all times. I can't say enough about it. It's a crazy-good kraut recipe, if I do say so myself.

Makes 2 quarts; 32 ¼-cup servings

¼ teaspoon Cutting Edge Starter Culture plus ½ cup water, or ¼ cup Kefir Whey (page 57)

1 small head cabbage (about 1 pound)

1 apple, unpeeled and cored

1 tablespoon Celtic Sea Salt

1 orange

If using the starter culture, stir together the culture and water. Let the mixture sit while you prepare the other ingredients—around 10 minutes.

Remove and discard the outer leaves of the cabbage. Finely shred the cabbage and apple, using a food processor or a hand shredder.

Mix the salt with the cabbage and apple.

Slice the orange into thin slices. Line the inside of the jar with orange slices or just layer them in the jar anywhere.

Pack the cabbage and apple mixture into the jar.

Add the starter culture or the whey and fill the jar with filtered water, leaving 2 to 3 inches of headspace to let the kraut bubble and expand as it ferments.

Seal the container and let it sit on your kitchen counter, out of direct sunlight, for 6 days.

Check the kraut every day to make sure it is fully submerged. If it has risen above the water, simply push it down so it is fully covered again. If white spots of yeast have formed on any unsubmerged kraut, do not worry. Remember, this isn't harmful. Just scoop out the yeast and kraut it's on and push the rest back under the water. (See FAQs on page 69 for more information.)

When the kraut is done fermenting, place it in the refrigerator.

Storage note: This kraut can be kept in an airtight jar in the refrigerator for up to 9 months.

KOMBUCHA BREAD

This is a unique way to have wonderful-tasting probiotic bread. Kombucha has the powerful probiotic yeast *Saccharomyces boulardii.* This is not the yeast that causes infections or overgrowth. *S. boulardii* exerts the opposite effect, producing lactic and other acids known to inhibit potentially harmful candida yeast species. And since this probiotic yeast is resistant to heat, you will actually receive more probiotics than you can in any other bread.

Makes 1 loaf; 8 servings

3 cups sprouted flour

1½ tablespoons baking powder

1 teaspoon Celtic Sea Salt

2 cups Basic Kombucha (page 62)

⅓ cup coconut sugar

Mix all the ingredients together in a large bowl, just until combined. Cover the bowl with a towel and let the dough sit for 5 to 7 hours. Bubbles and cracks will form in the dough.

Preheat the oven to 350°F and lightly grease a 9 x 5-inch loaf pan.

Transfer the dough to the loaf pan and bake for 55 minutes.

Remove the bread from the oven and allow it to cool in the pan for about 5 minutes. Then remove the bread from the pan, place it on a cooling rack, and serve it while it's still warm.

KOMBUCHA PICKLES

My daughter Maci has a love affair with kombucha, and many of the kombucha recipes in this book are from her. She makes gallons of it. One day she decided to play around with culturing vegetables using kombucha, and this superfast pickle recipe was the result. One note: You need to eat these within a week as they can get mushy beyond that point. This is due to the different culture we are using. Don't be surprised when you taste these; they have a milder flavor than your average pickle.

Makes 1 quart; 7 to 10 servings

7 to 10 mini pickling cucumbers, enough to fill your jar

2 teaspoons Celtic Sea Salt

2 teaspoons dill

½ teaspoon dried mustard

½ teaspoon pepper

½ teaspoon chili powder

Kombucha to fill the jar

....

Add the cucumbers and spices to the jar.

Fill the jar with kombucha, leaving 2 to 3 inches of headspace to let the pickles bubble and expand as they ferment.

Seal the container and let it sit on your kitchen counter, out of direct sunlight, for 2 days.

Check the pickles each day to make sure they are fully submerged in the kombucha. If they have risen above the kombucha, simply flip them over and push them down so they are fully covered.

The pickles will change color as they ferment. Once they do, refrigerate them.

Storage note: These pickles can be kept in an airtight jar in the refrigerator for up to 1 week.

FERMENTED CUCUMBER TOMATO SALAD

I've made this delicious salad for many a party. I especially love to prepare it in the summer because summer tomatoes make this dish extra delicious. Sometimes I add more fresh, unfermented tomatoes to stretch the dish to feed more people. In my mind, the more tomatoes the merrier!

Makes 1 quart; 16 ¼-cup servings

For the veggies

⅛ teaspoon Cutting Edge Starter Culture plus ¼ cup water, or 2 tablespoons Kefir Whey (page 57)

3 medium tomatoes

¼ red onion

1 cucumber

2 teaspoons Celtic Sea Salt

¼ teaspoon coarse ground pepper

For the salad

¼ cup finely chopped fresh parsley

Olive oil for drizzling

⅓ cup crumbled feta cheese (optional)

A few black olives, sliced (optional)

....

If using the starter culture, stir together the culture and water. Let the mixture sit while you prepare the other ingredients—around 10 minutes.

Cut the tomatoes in half lengthwise and remove the seeds. Then thinly slice the tomatoes.

Peel the onion and slice it thinly.

Halve the cucumber and slice it into small chunks.

Place the tomatoes, onion, cucumbers, salt, and pepper in a large bowl and toss to combine.

Transfer the mixture to your jar and add the starter culture or the whey. Then fill the jar with filtered water, leaving 2 to 3 inches of headspace to let the veggies bubble and expand as they ferment.

Seal the container and let it sit on your kitchen counter, out of direct sunlight, for 2 days.

Check the vegetables every day to make sure they are fully submerged. If they have risen above the water, simply push them down so they are fully covered again. If white spots of yeast have formed on any unsubmerged vegetables, do not worry. Remember, this isn't harmful. Just scoop out the yeast and vegetables it's on and push the rest back under the water. (See FAQs on page 69 for more information.)

After 2 days, scoop out the vegetables with a slotted spoon and place them in a bowl.

Toss with parsley and drizzle with olive oil. Add feta and olives if desired.

Serve immediately.

MEXICAN CARROTS

My son is an auto mechanic, and he often gets delicious Mexican food from a woman who comes into his shop on a regular basis. She brought him a canned version of these carrots, but, of course, when I re-created the recipe, I fermented it. The flavors are amazing and it's super spicy! If you want it milder, simply take the seeds out of the jalapeños before fermenting.

Makes 1 quart; 16 ¼-cup servings

⅛ teaspoon Cutting Edge Starter Culture plus ¼ cup water, or 2 tablespoons Kefir Whey (page 57)

4 carrots

1 small jalapeño pepper

1 clove garlic

1 bay leaf

1 tablespoon black peppercorns

½ teaspoon Celtic Sea Salt

....

If using the starter culture, stir together the culture and water. Let the mixture sit while you prepare the other ingredients—around 10 minutes.

Peel the carrots and slice them on the diagonal.

Slice the jalapeño into thin pieces.

Mince the garlic.

Place the carrots, jalapeño, garlic, bay leaf, peppercorns, and salt in a bowl and mix to combine.

Transfer the mixture to your jar and add the starter culture or the whey. Then fill the jar with filtered water, leaving 2 to 3 inches of headspace to let the carrots bubble and expand as they ferment.

Seal the container and let it sit on your kitchen counter, out of direct sunlight, for 3 days.

Check the carrots every day to make sure they are fully submerged. If they have risen above the water, simply push them down so they are fully covered again. If white spots of yeast have formed on any unsubmerged carrots, do not worry. Remember, this isn't harmful. Just scoop out the yeast and carrots it's on and push the rest back under the water. (See FAQs on page 69 for more information.)

When the carrots are done fermenting, place them in the refrigerator.

Storage note: These carrots can be kept in an airtight jar in the refrigerator for up to 9 months.

BLUEBERRY SPINACH KRAUT

If you like blueberries, you will love this kraut. I enjoy it most after it has been in the fridge for a few weeks. It gets better with age, and at four to five weeks it's super tasty.

Makes 2 quarts; 32 ¼-cup servings

¼ teaspoon Cutting Edge Starter Culture plus ½ cup water, or ¼ cup Kefir Whey (page 57)

½ head green cabbage

1 large shallot

1 tablespoon organic Herbamare seasoning or Celtic Sea Salt

1 cup chopped or shredded spinach

1½ cups fresh blueberries

½ cup 100% fruit cranberry or blueberry juice

....

If using the starter culture, stir together the culture and water. Let the mixture sit while you prepare the other ingredients—around 10 minutes.

Remove and discard the outer leaves of the cabbage. Shred or finely chop the cabbage and the shallot. Place the cabbage in a bowl and sprinkle it with Herbamare seasoning.

Then add the shallot, spinach, and blueberries and toss to combine.

Firmly pack the mixture into two 1-quart jars.

Add half the culture or kefir whey and half the juice to each jar. Then fill the containers with filtered water, leaving 2 to 3 inches of headspace to let the kraut bubble and expand as it ferments.

Seal the containers and let them sit on your kitchen counter, out of direct sunlight, for 6 days.

Check the kraut every day to make sure it is fully submerged. If it has risen above the water, simply push it down so it is fully covered again. If white spots of yeast have formed on any unsubmerged kraut, do not worry. Remember, this isn't harmful. Just scoop out the yeast and kraut it's on and push the rest back under the water. (See FAQs on page 69 for more information.)

When the kraut is done fermenting, place it in the refrigerator.

Storage note: This kraut can be kept in an airtight jar in the refrigerator for up to 9 months.

SALAD IN A FERMENTING JAR

This recipe is my new obsession. I love to pack it in a cooler—with a bunch of other fermented foods—and take it along when we go to the lake on the weekends. When I don't take my cultures and cultured foods, I feel as if I am leaving my kids at home alone. It would just be wrong not to bring them!

Makes 1 serving

10 Cultured Italian Tomato halves (page 136)

5 thinly sliced rings purple onion

6 dried apple chips

2 handfuls spinach

3 tablespoons blue cheese crumbles

1/3 cup chopped pecans

2 tablespoons Apple Kefir Dressing (page 190)

Layer all ingredients in a jar in order, starting with the tomatoes on the bottom and topping off with the pecans.

Top with Apple Kefir Dressing immediately before eating.

You can eat this right away, or cap and place in the refrigerator until you're ready to eat. It is best to eat this within 1 day.

CULTURED ZUCCHINI AND YAMS

This is perfect for the holidays, served as a side dish or alongside a sweet potato casserole. It is also delicious served on top of a baked yam. But honestly, I eat it with a spoon straight from the jar.

Makes 2 quarts; 32 ¼-cup servings

¼ teaspoon Cutting Edge Starter Culture plus ½ cup water, or ¼ cup Kefir Whey (page 57)

2 large zucchini

2 large yams

1 small onion

2 teaspoons salt

⅓ cup apple juice

If using the starter culture, stir together the culture and water. Let the mixture sit while you prepare the other ingredients—around 10 minutes.

Shred the zucchini, yams, and onion, using a food processor or a hand shredder.

Place the vegetables together in a bowl, add salt, and toss to mix.

Transfer the mixture to your jar and add the apple juice and the starter culture or the whey. Then fill the jar with filtered water, leaving 2 to 3 inches of headspace to let the veggies bubble and expand as they ferment.

Seal the container and let it sit on your kitchen counter, out of direct sunlight, for 2 days.

Check the vegetables every day to make sure they are fully submerged. If they have risen above the water, simply push them down so they are fully covered again. If white spots of yeast have formed on unsubmerged vegetables, do not worry. Remember, this isn't harmful. Just scoop out the yeast and vegetables it's on and push the rest back under the water. (See FAQs on page 69 for more information.)

When the veggies are done fermenting, place them in the refrigerator.

Storage note: These veggies can be kept in an airtight jar in the refrigerator for up to 9 months.

THE FAIREST KALE SALAD IN THE LAND

This is the best kale salad I've ever had. I love the taste of the toasted nuts and seeds, and the cultured dressing is to die for. Plus it incorporates two parts of the Trilogy. I hope you enjoy it as much as I do!

Makes 5 servings

1 cup pecan halves

½ cup sesame seeds (optional)

1 medium bunch kale, stemmed and finely chopped

3 cups baby spinach, chopped

3 cloves garlic, quartered

¼ cup Kefir Cheese (page 57)

¼ cup Basic Kefir (page 51)

1 tablespoon Basic Kombucha (page 62)

½ lemon, juiced and zested

3 tablespoons olive oil

¼ teaspoon Celtic Sea Salt

1½ tablespoons nutritional yeast

1 small apple, cored and chopped finely

....

Preheat the oven to 300°F.

Place pecans and sesame seeds, if using, on a baking sheet and toast in the oven until they are lightly browned, about 8 minutes.

Meanwhile, toss the kale and spinach in a large salad bowl and set aside.

Put the garlic, kefir cheese, kefir, kombucha, lemon juice and zest, 2 tablespoons of the olive oil, and the salt in a food processor or blender. Process until combined.

Drizzle this mixture over the kale and spinach and toss to combine.

Place the toasted pecans and sesame seeds in a food processor along with the nutritional yeast, the remaining 1 tablespoon of olive oil, and a pinch of salt. Pulse until the mixture is the size of small peas.

Sprinkle the pecan mixture and the apple over the kale and spinach mixture. Toss again to combine.

This is best when eaten immediately, but it can be stored in the fridge for a few hours before serving.

CULTURED BROCCOLI SALAD IN A JAR

Broccoli isn't the first thing people think of when looking for something to ferment, but I say this salad is to die for—and not just the salad, the juice, too! The grapes and raisins add sweetness while the onion gives it a little kick. Trust me; it's delicious.

Makes 2 quarts; 32 ¼-cup servings

¼ teaspoon Cutting Edge Starter Culture plus ½ cup water, or ¼ cup Kefir Whey (page 57)

1 head broccoli, florets only

2 medium carrots

1 small red onion

½ cup raisins

½ cup grapes

2 teaspoons lemon juice, freshly squeezed

1½ teaspoons Celtic Sea Salt

....

If using the starter culture, stir together the culture and water. Let the mixture sit while you prepare the other ingredients—around 10 minutes.

Chop the broccoli and place in a large bowl.

Shred the carrots, using a food processor or hand shredder, and thinly slice the onion. Add the carrots, onion, raisins, grapes, lemon juice, and salt to the broccoli. Stir to combine.

Transfer the mixture to your jar and add the starter culture or the whey. Then fill the jar with filtered water, leaving 2 to 3 inches of headspace to let the veggies bubble and expand as they ferment.

Seal the container and let it sit on your kitchen counter, out of direct sunlight, for 3 days.

Check the vegetables every day to make sure they are fully submerged. If they have risen above the water, simply push them down so they fully covered again. If white spots of yeast have formed on unsubmerged vegetables, do not worry. Remember, this isn't harmful. Just scoop out the yeast and vegetables it's on and push the rest back under the water. (See FAQs on page 69 for more information.)

When the veggies are done fermenting, place them in the refrigerator.

Storage note: These veggies can be kept in an airtight jar in the refrigerator for up to 9 months.

CULTURED RED AND YELLOW PEPPERS

These peppers are so handy to have around. You can use them on salads, in dips and salsas, as a pizza topping, and so on—just scoop them out of the jar and use them anywhere you would use fresh peppers. You'll find tons of uses for them, and if nothing else, they look really pretty culturing on the counter.

Makes 1 quart; 16 ¼-cup servings

⅛ teaspoon Cutting Edge Starter Culture plus ¼ cup water, or 2 tablespoons Kefir Whey (page 57)

2 red bell peppers

1 yellow bell pepper

1 clove garlic (optional)

1 tablespoon mustard seeds

1 tablespoon Celtic Sea Salt

....

If using the starter culture, stir together the culture and water. Let the mixture sit while you prepare the other ingredients—around 10 minutes.

Cut the peppers in half and remove the pith, seeds, and stems. Then cut into half-inch slices.

Place peppers, garlic (if using), mustard seeds, and salt into a jar.

Add the starter culture or the whey. Then fill the jar with filtered water, leaving 2 to 3 inches of headspace to let the peppers bubble and expand as they ferment.

Seal the container and let it sit on your kitchen counter, out of direct sunlight, for 3 days.

Check the peppers every day to make sure they are fully submerged. If they have risen above the water, simply push them down so they are fully covered again. If white spots of yeast have formed on any unsubmerged peppers, do not worry. Remember, this isn't harmful. Just scoop out the yeast and peppers it's on and push the rest back under the water. (See FAQs on page 69 for more information.)

When the peppers are done fermenting, place them in the refrigerator.

Storage note: These peppers can be kept in an airtight jar in the refrigerator for up to 9 months.

CULTURED CARROT CAKE IN A JAR

You probably think of carrot cake as a dessert—and for the most part, you're right. But this recipe might change your mind. It uses all healthy ingredients, so you can serve it as a side dish, but people will believe they're eating a sweet treat. I eat this when I want to feel like I'm being bad.

Makes 1 quart; 16 ¼-cup servings

2 carrots, peeled and shredded

2 apples, cored and shredded

4 dates, chopped

⅛ cup chopped walnuts

⅛ teaspoon nutmeg

⅛ teaspoon cloves

½ teaspoon cinnamon

½ teaspoon Celtic Sea Salt

½ teaspoon vanilla

¼ teaspoon Cutting Edge Starter Culture

....

Combine the carrots, apples, dates, and walnuts in a bowl and stir to mix.

Add the nutmeg, cloves, cinnamon, salt, and vanilla and stir until evenly incorporated.

Transfer the mixture to a jar and sprinkle it with the starter culture. Then fill the jar with filtered water, leaving 2 to 3 inches of headspace to let the veggies bubble and expand as they ferment.

Seal the container and let it sit on your kitchen counter, out of direct sunlight, for 2 to 3 days. When it's ready, the carrots and apples should still be firm but a bit tart.

Check the mixture every day to make sure the carrots and apples are fully submerged. If they have risen above the water, simply push them down so they are fully covered again. If white spots of yeast have formed on any unsubmerged pieces, do not worry. Remember, this isn't harmful. Just scoop out the yeast and carrot or apple pieces it's on and push the rest back under the water. (See FAQs on page 69 for more information.)

When the mixture is done fermenting, place it in the refrigerator.

Storage note: This can be kept in an airtight jar in the refrigerator for up to 3 months.

CULTURED APPLE PIE IN A JAR

I've had quite a few people ask me if you can ferment fruit. The answer is yes, you certainly can! Just remember that the good bacteria eat the sugars out of the fruit, so it does get a little tart, and the tartness intensifies over time. That's why I like to eat cultured fruits right away.

Makes 1 quart; 16 ¼-cup servings

4 apples

¼ teaspoon cinnamon

⅛ teaspoon nutmeg

½ teaspoon Celtic Sea Salt

½ teaspoon vanilla

¼ teaspoon Cutting Edge Starter Culture

....

Core and shred the apples.

Combine the apples, cinnamon, nutmeg, salt, and vanilla in a small bowl and mix with a spoon or your hands.

Transfer the mixture to a jar and sprinkle it with the starter culture.

Fill the jar with filtered water, leaving 2 to 3 inches of headspace to let the fruit bubble and expand as it ferments.

Seal the container and let it sit on your kitchen counter, out of direct sunlight, for 3 days.

Check the fruit every day to make sure it is fully submerged. If it has risen above the water, simply push it down so it is fully covered again. If white spots of yeast have formed on any unsubmerged apple, do not worry. Remember, this isn't harmful. Just scoop out the yeast and fruit it's on and push the rest back under the water. (See FAQs on page 69 for more information.)

Once it's ready, place it in the refrigerator.

Storage note: This can be kept in an airtight jar in the refrigerator for up to 3 months.

CHAPTER 11

Desserts

COCONUT KEFIR GRAHAMS

My 13-year-old daughter Holli took these coconut grahams to class one day. One thing led to another, and soon some of the moms discovered that Holli was my daughter. These moms had been to my classes, bought my book, and had been making cultured foods. Excitedly, they asked Holli if they could try her grahams. Of course she shared. And when she got home, she said, "They think you're famous. So I turned down all the treats and sweets at class because I want to be an example, too. And since I had the grahams, I didn't even want the other stuff anyway." That's my girl. ☺

Makes 12 servings

For the graham crackers

2 cups sprouted whole wheat flour

¼ teaspoon Celtic Sea Salt

¼ teaspoon baking soda

¼ teaspoon baking powder

5 tablespoons melted butter

4 tablespoons honey

2 to 4 tablespoons water

For the topping

1 small zucchini, peeled and cubed

¾ cup coconut milk

2 teaspoons vanilla

1 cup Coconut Kefir Cheese (page 59)

2 cups shredded coconut

½ cup pine nuts

¼ cup coconut oil, melted

Honey or stevia to taste

....

Preheat the oven to 350°F.

Grease a large baking sheet or line it with parchment paper.

To make the grahams, mix together the flour, salt, baking soda, and baking powder in a large bowl.

Add the butter, honey, and just enough water to form a ball that is not sticky to the touch.

Roll out the dough directly onto the prepared baking sheet.

Score the dough into 12 crackers with a sharp knife, then prick the dough all over with a fork.

Bake the crackers for 20 to 25 minutes.

Transfer the crackers, still in the pan, to a wire rack to cool completely.

For the topping, put the zucchini, coconut milk, and vanilla in a food processor and pulse until smooth.

Add the kefir cheese, coconut, and pine nuts to the zucchini mixture and pulse until thoroughly combined and smooth.

Add the coconut oil and pulse again a few times until combined.

Refrigerate for 1 to 3 hours or until the mixture thickens.

When you're ready to eat these, simply scoop the topping onto the graham crackers.

Storage note: The crackers can be stored in a sealed container in your cabinet for 2 weeks. The coconut mixture can be kept in an airtight jar in the refrigerator for up to 3 days.

CHOCOLATE KEFIR CANDY

I keep chocolate kefir candy in the freezer or fridge pretty much all the time, so we can have a little chocolate when we need something sweet and decadent. The candies are small but rich in nutrients, so one can satisfy you.

Makes 24 servings

24 mini cupcake liners

2 cups chocolate chips or bars, 60% to 70% cacao

½ cup shredded coconut

½ cup pine nuts

1 cup Kefir Cheese (page 57)

Zest of one orange

8 packages stevia or 2 tablespoons honey

....

Place the mini cupcake liners in mini muffin pans.

Melt 1 cup of the chocolate in a double boiler, stirring constantly. Remove the chocolate from the heat and add ¼ cup of coconut and ¼ cup of pine nuts. Mix to combine.

Drop 1 tablespoon of the mixture into each muffin cup, then place these in the freezer.

Mix the kefir cheese, orange zest, and stevia in a small bowl.

When chocolate is frozen, remove the muffin tin from the freezer and spread ½ tablespoon of the kefir cheese mixture on top of the chocolate.

Put the muffin tin in the fridge.

Melt the remaining 1 cup of chocolate in a double boiler, stirring constantly. Remove the chocolate from the heat and add the remaining ¼ cup of coconut and ¼ cup of pine nuts, mixing to combine. Let the chocolate cool until it's warm but not hot, about 5 to 10 minutes.

Remove the muffin tin from the refrigerator and spread the chocolate on top of the kefir cheese.

Place the candies in the refrigerator until solid, about 1 hour.

RAW KEFIR PUMPKIN PIE

If you like pumpkin pie, you're going to love this recipe. My family said this is the best dessert I have made, and it lasts only about a day in my house. It is a raw dessert, and the crust is a snap to make. And the flavor? Well . . . it is a wow!

Makes 8 servings

For the crust

1 cup walnuts

1 cup pecans

1 cup raisins

Pinch Celtic Sea Salt

For the filling

1 cup raw cashews, soaked for 3 to 4 hours in water and then drained

1 cup pumpkin puree

1 cup Kefir Cheese (page 57)

½ cup maple syrup

½ cup coconut oil, melted

2 teaspoons vanilla

1 teaspoon cinnamon

⅛ teaspoon Celtic Sea Salt

⅛ teaspoon ground ginger

¼ teaspoon nutmeg

1 cup Coconut Whipped Cream (page 179)

To make the crust, pulse the walnuts and pecans in a food processor until they're crumbs, then add the raisins and salt and pulse until the mixture begins to stick together.

Press the mixture into a pie dish and put it in the fridge.

For the filling, combine the cashews, pumpkin, kefir cheese, maple syrup, coconut oil, vanilla, cinnamon, salt, ginger, and nutmeg in a blender or food processor on high speed. Pulse until completely smooth. This can take a few minutes.

Pour the filling into the crust, then cover it with plastic wrap.

Place the pie in the freezer until solid, about 5 hours. Before slicing and serving, let the pie sit at room temperature for 10 minutes to soften a little.

Top with Coconut Whipped Cream before serving.

APPLE PIE PARFAIT

I gave up sugar right before my daughter's wedding. We didn't eat it all that much, but I decided to burn the bridge and call it quits, which is why a lot of my recipes use stevia. I really don't crave sugar anymore, and if I need something sweet, I make things like this to satisfy myself. This recipe was inspired by a feast at a friend's house last Thanksgiving. Everybody was eating apple pie, and the smell of apples and cinnamon filled the house. I came up with this to make my house smell amazing, too.

Makes 1 serving

1 cup cooked quinoa or oatmeal, chilled

1 apple, cored and sliced thinly

¾ cup Kefir Cheese (page 57)

¼ cup honey or 3 packages stevia

¼ teaspoon cinnamon

2 tablespoons chopped walnuts

Preheat the oven to 350ºF.

Spread the apple slices in the bottom of a small baking dish. Add two tablespoons of water to the baking dish and bake the apples for 15 minutes or until tender. Remove them from the oven and let them cool for approximately 10 minutes.

Mix together the kefir cheese, honey, cinnamon, and quinoa or oatmeal in a small bowl.

Layer half of the kefir cheese mixture in the bottom of a glass jar, followed by 1 tablespoon of the walnuts and half the apples. Repeat the layers to create a parfait.

Serve immediately or store in the refrigerator for up to 3 days.

OVERNIGHT KEFIR BROWNIE PUDDING

The first time I made this yummy concoction, I walked around my house asking my family to try it. I got the same response from everybody: "Mmm, that's really good! Tastes like a brownie." Hence the name. If you have picky eaters in your house who refuse to try kefir, this will help convert them. Just don't tell them they're eating kefir until after they've tried it. I always tell people that if they hang around me long enough, eventually they will be converted. Resistance is futile.

Makes 2 servings

¾ cup unsweetened almond milk

½ cup Basic Kefir (page 51)

2 tablespoons cocoa powder

2 packages stevia or 2 tablespoons maple syrup

¾ cup raw old-fashioned oatmeal (also called rolled oats)

2 tablespoons shredded coconut

2 tablespoons chopped almonds

Mix together the almond milk, kefir, cocoa powder, stevia, and oatmeal in a 1-quart canning jar.

Seal the jar and refrigerate overnight.

Before eating, top with the coconut and almonds.

LEMON KEFIR CANDY

The coconut cream concentrate used in this recipe is different from coconut milk or oil. It is similar to the milk, but it contains some of the flesh of the coconut, which makes for a different consistency, thicker and more paste-like. You can find coconut cream concentrate in most health food stores or online. It makes yummy treats and desserts.

Makes 12 servings

½ cup coconut cream concentrate

½ cup Kefir Cheese (page 57)

½ cup honey

Juice and zest of ½ lemon

½ cup shredded coconut

2 tablespoons psyllium husk

....

Mix together all of the ingredients in a medium bowl.

Spoon the mixture in bite-size portions onto a cookie sheet, using a small cookie scoop. Then refrigerate overnight until completely solidified.

KEFIR COCONUT RUM BALLS

Why do we eat so much junk food at the holidays? It's a habit and a choice, and just as you trained yourself to eat unhealthy foods, you can learn to substitute healthy options that are just as delicious and easy to make and reach for. If you have healthy treats around, like these rum balls, you will eat them. Plus, you can make them in a snap and freeze them for later.

Makes 40 servings

2 cups almond flour

1 cup finely shredded coconut

½ cup Basic Kefir (page 51)

2 tablespoons psyllium husk

¼ cup honey

2 teaspoons vanilla

¼ cup cocoa powder

¾ cup coconut oil, melted but not hot

2 tablespoons light rum or 1 teaspoon rum extract

½ cup chopped walnuts*

....

Line a cookie sheet with parchment paper.

Combine the almond flour, coconut, kefir, psyllium husk, honey, vanilla, cocoa powder, coconut oil, and rum (if using) in a medium mixing bowl. Stir until thoroughly combined.

Using a small cookie scoop, spoon the batter onto the cookie sheet in bite-size balls.

Refrigerate the balls for 5 to 10 minutes, then roll them in the walnuts.

Refrigerate until firm; eat within a couple of days.

*You can make these with any coating you want. I've used different kinds of nuts, coconut, cranberries, goji berries, cocoa powder—and so much more! Use whatever tastes good to you.

SUPERFAST BANANA KEFIR ICE CREAM

This is one of my very favorite desserts, and I want it all the time—especially in the warm summer months. Consequently, I always keep chopped bananas in the freezer. Then I can have this dessert ready in minutes.

Makes 1 serving

1 frozen chopped banana*

¼ cup Basic Kefir (page 51)

½ teaspoon cinnamon

1 teaspoon honey or ¼ teaspoon stevia

....

Place the frozen banana pieces in a food processor and pulse until the banana looks crumbly or smashed. Scrape down the food processor.

Add the kefir, cinnamon, and honey and pulse until the mixture looks creamy, like ice cream.

Serve immediately or transfer to an airtight container and freeze for up to 1 month.

*Make sure to peel and chop the banana before you freeze it!

TROPICAL KEFIR PUDDING

This is a recipe I served at my Camp Trilogy Class. My husband and daughter came to help me pass it out in sample cups, and my husband, bless his heart, served it with sprouted corn chips instead of the spoons I had brought. I noticed the surprised look on people's faces as they scooped up this fruity pudding with a corn chip. I had to laugh; he would serve corn chips with everything if he could. However, this is best served with extra fruit, not corn chips!

Makes 4 servings

2 avocados

1 mango

1 kiwi

1 cup Basic Kefir (page 51)

2 tablespoons lime juice

2 teaspoons lime zest

½ teaspoon lemon extract

¼ teaspoon Celtic Sea Salt

2 to 3 teaspoons stevia powder, or 2 to 3 tablespoons Sucanat or honey

1 tablespoon chia seeds

Toasted shredded coconut (optional)

Cut the avocados, mango, and kiwi in half and scoop the fruit out of the skins.

Combine the fruit and the kefir, lime juice and zest, lemon extract, salt, stevia, and chia seeds in a blender or food processor. Process until smooth and thick like pudding.

Separate the mixture into four bowls and chill for at least 30 minutes before serving.

Top with toasted coconut if desired.

CHOCOLATE KEFIR COCONUT PUDDING

This dairy-free pudding is crazy good and a huge hit at my classes. I mean, who doesn't love chocolate and coconut?

Makes 1 serving

1 cup Coconut Kefir (page 59)

2 teaspoons cocoa powder

1 tablespoon chia seeds

1 teaspoon vanilla

Stevia, honey, or Sucanat to taste

Whisk together the coconut kefir, cocoa powder, chia seeds, vanilla, and stevia until well combined.

Transfer the mixture to a 1-pint jar. Secure the lid and place the jar in the fridge.

Refrigerate until the mixture is thick and creamy, at least 3 hours.

STRAWBERRY KEFIR ICE CREAM

This is my daughter Holli's favorite kefir ice cream. While you can make it with almond milk or regular milk, I like to use canned coconut milk because it gives the ice cream such a rich and decadent consistency.

Makes 4 servings

1⅓ cups Second-Fermented Citrus Kefir, made with lemon (page 56)

1 cup Kefir Cheese (page 57)

1½ cups coconut milk

1 cup fresh strawberries, hulled

½ cup honey, Sucanat, or coconut sugar

1 to 2 leaves fresh basil (optional)

. . . .

Place all the ingredients, except the basil, in the blender and blend for about 1 minute.

Taste the mixture and add more sweetener, if desired, until it tastes good to you.

Pour the mixture into an ice cream maker and process according to the manufacturer's instructions.

Top with fresh basil, if desired, before serving.

COCONUT ALMOND KEFIR ICE CREAM

I just can't get over how delicious kefir ice cream is. It's smooth and creamy, and it's packed with healthy probiotics. I love that I can create a healthy gut while enjoying a delicious treat.

Makes 4 servings

1 cup Coconut Kefir Cheese (page 59)

3 cups almond or coconut milk, or a combination of the two

1 teaspoon vanilla

½ cup honey, Sucanat, or coconut sugar

1 cup shredded coconut

Place the kefir cheese, milk, vanilla, and sweetener in a blender and mix for 15 to 20 seconds.

Taste the mixture and add more sweetener, if desired, until it tastes good to you.

Pour the mixture into an ice cream maker and process according to the manufacturer's instructions.

About 10 minutes before you plan to serve the ice cream, preheat the oven to 400°F.

Spread the shredded coconut on a baking sheet and bake until it is toasted brown, about 5 minutes.

Sprinkle the ice cream with toasted coconut.

BERRY KOMBUCHA MIXER

Do you want a treat that will pick you up and make you feel great? I make this kombucha all the time, especially in the summer, when berries are abundant. It's so easy to make that you could argue that it's barely even a recipe, but I wanted to include it because it hits the spot every time.

Makes 1 serving

1½ cups mixed berries

1 cup Basic Kombucha (page 62)

Place the berries in a large glass. Pour the kombucha over the top and serve with a large spoon.

CHAPTER 12

Beverages

PEACH KOMBUCHA SANGRIA

This is my daughter Maci's recipe. She recently got married and spent her honeymoon in Laguna Beach, California, and came home inspired by all the fresh-fruit drinks they had. For this recipe we use fresh peaches from our tree in the backyard. I like to add a splash of vanilla because peaches and vanilla are heavenly together.

Makes 2 servings

½ cup chopped fresh peaches

2 cups Basic Kombucha (page 62)

1 teaspoon Sucanat or sugar

½ teaspoon vanilla (optional)

Place all the ingredients in a mason jar with a lid (plastic is preferable).

Let the kombucha sit on your kitchen counter for two days. Then strain the peaches and serve the kombucha, or store it in the refrigerator.

Storage note: This kombucha will last in the sealed container in the fridge for 1 year but will turn to vinegar over time. It is fine to drink but might be better used as vinegar because of the sour taste. Once open, the carbonation will start to decrease—just as with regular store-bought soda.

KOMBUCHA UTI BUSTER

WebMD reports that if you drink cranberry juice, within eight hours the levels of bad bacteria in the urinary tract decrease; thus, cranberry juice could prevent an infection. If you're fighting a urinary tract infection, try this drink. The healing properties of cranberry juice plus the good bacteria of kombucha make for a powerful combination. You won't believe how fast it can work and how simple it is to prepare.

Makes 1 serving

½ cup fresh, whole cranberries

2 cups Basic Kombucha (page 62) or Second-Fermented Kombucha (page 64)

½ cup ice

½ dropperful liquid stevia (optional)

....

Place all the ingredients in a blender and process until well blended. Serve immediately.

CRANBERRY LIME KOMBUCHA SPARKLER

My daughter Maci is lovingly referred to by her friends as the kombucha queen—and deservedly so. Almost all the kombucha recipes in this book came from her. She makes kombucha much more often than I do. When she prepares this recipe, I beg her to make some for me. It's so refreshing that I just can't get enough of it.

Makes 16 ounces; 1 serving

1¾ cups Basic Kombucha (page 62)

¼ cup unsweetened cranberry juice

1 tablespoon lime juice

Place all the ingredients in a sturdy bottle, leaving a little headspace at the top.

Clamp the cap closed and date the bottle so you know when the second fermentation began.

Let the kombucha sit on your kitchen counter, out of direct sunlight, for 1 to 3 weeks.

Check the kombucha after each week to see if it is bubbly enough for you. If not, let it ferment longer.

Once the kombucha suits your taste, transfer the bottle to the refrigerator.

Storage note: This kombucha will last in the sealed container in the fridge for 1 year but will turn to vinegar over time. It is still fine to drink but might be better used as vinegar because of the sour taste. Once open, the carbonation will start to decrease—just as with regular store-bought soda.

GINGER KOMBUCHA

This is one of the most popular kombucha recipes—easy to make and oh so good for you. Ginger provides a very earthy flavor with a little bit of a bite to it. I love the taste of fresh ginger, and it makes kombucha really bubbly.

Makes 16 ounces; 1 serving

1¾ cups Basic Kombucha (page 62)

2-inch piece fresh ginger

1 long strip lemon peel

Place all the ingredients in a sturdy bottle, leaving a little headspace at the top.

Clamp the cap closed and date the bottle so you know when the second fermentation began.

Let the kombucha sit on your kitchen counter, out of direct sunlight, for 1 to 3 weeks.

Check the kombucha after each week to see if it is bubbly enough for you. If not, let it ferment longer.

Once the kombucha suits your taste, transfer the bottle to the refrigerator.

Storage note: This kombucha will last in the sealed container in the fridge for 1 year but will turn to vinegar over time. It is still fine to drink but might be better used as vinegar because of the sour taste. Once open, the carbonation will start to decrease—just as with regular store-bought soda.

COUGH-BUSTER KOMBUCHA

Pineapples contain bromelain, an enzyme with anti-inflammatory properties. The juice from fresh pineapples can suppress coughs five times more effectively than cough syrup. Drinking pineapple juice with kombucha can help heal a sore throat while also helping the body expel mucus. My family knows that whenever they have a sore throat, I will tell them to drink kombucha. Most people reach for medicine and lozenges, but we always reach for this kombucha.

Makes 16 ounces; 1 serving

1¾ cups Basic Kombucha (page 62)

¼ cup pineapple juice

½ tablespoon honey

Place all the ingredients in a sturdy bottle, leaving a little headspace at the top.

Clamp the cap closed and date the bottle so you know when the second fermentation began.

Let the kombucha sit on your kitchen counter, out of direct sunlight, for 1 to 3 weeks.

Check the kombucha after each week to see if it is bubbly enough for you. If not, let it ferment longer.

Once the kombucha suits your taste, transfer the bottle to the refrigerator.

Storage note: This kombucha will last in the sealed container in the fridge for 1 year but will turn to vinegar over time. It is still fine to drink but might be better used as vinegar because of the sour taste. Once open, the carbonation will start to decrease—just as with regular store-bought soda.

GINGERBREAD KOMBUCHA

The unique gingerbread taste in this kombucha comes from molasses. There are many types of molasses on the market; for this recipe, make sure to use organic blackstrap molasses. It has many health benefits that have been refined out of other types of molasses, including high amounts of copper, calcium, magnesium, and iron. Plus it's loaded with B vitamins that make your hair and nails beautiful and strong.

Makes 16 ounces; 1 serving

1¾ cups Basic Kombucha (page 62)

1 tablespoon organic blackstrap molasses

1 cinnamon stick

Place all the ingredients in a sturdy bottle, leaving a little headspace at the top.

Clamp the cap closed and date the bottle so you know when the second fermentation began.

Let the kombucha sit on your kitchen counter, out of direct sunlight, for 1 to 3 weeks.

Check the kombucha after each week to see if it is bubbly enough for you. If not, let it ferment longer.

Once the kombucha suits your taste, transfer the bottle to the refrigerator.

Storage note: This kombucha will last in the sealed container in the fridge for 1 year but will turn to vinegar over time. It is still fine to drink but might be better used as vinegar because of the sour taste. Once open, the carbonation will start to decrease—just as with regular store-bought soda.

FIZZY BLENDER-JUICED APPLE KOMBUCHA

When you second-ferment kombucha using freshly squeezed juice rather than bottled or other premade juice, your kombucha will get fizzier faster because of all the enzymes in the fruit. And you don't need a juicer—you can make apple juice in your blender in a snap.

Makes 2 quarts; four servings

5 apples

7 cups Basic Kombucha (page 62)

....

Core the apples and cut them into slices.

Place the apple slices in a blender and add ½ cup water. Blend on high until the apples are liquefied.

Strain the apple juice by placing a coffee filter in a strainer, placing the strainer over a bowl, and pouring the apple juice into the strainer. Let it sit until all the juice has run through the strainer.

Mix the apple juice with the kombucha, then transfer the mixture into 4 bottles.

Seal the bottles and let the kombucha sit on your kitchen counter, out of direct sunlight, for 1 to 3 days. The fermentation time will depend on how sweet your kombucha was to start with and the temperature in your house.

Check the bottles often in order to taste the kombucha and to release the pressure. When the kombucha is bubbly, it is done.

Place the bottles in the refrigerator.

Storage note: This kombucha will last in the sealed containers in the fridge for 1 year but will turn to vinegar over time. It is still fine to drink but might be better used as vinegar because of the sour taste. Once open, the carbonation will start to decrease—just as with regular store-bought soda.

SUNSHINE KOMBUCHA

I aim to have carrots every day because of how good they are for your eyes. For quite a while I tried to figure out a good way to use them with kombucha, but I never liked the results—until now. I discovered that you can't just use carrot juice—you have to combine it with other juices. When I happened upon the combo of orange, pineapple, and carrot, what I found was divine! It tastes like sunshine!

Makes 16 ounces; 1 serving

1¾ cups Basic Kombucha (page 62)

2 tablespoons orange juice

2 tablespoons carrot juice

2 tablespoons pineapple juice

....

Place all the ingredients in a sturdy bottle, leaving a little headspace at the top.

Clamp the cap closed and date the bottle so you know when the second fermentation began.

Let the kombucha sit on your kitchen counter, out of direct sunlight, for 1 to 3 weeks.

Check the kombucha after each week to see if it is bubbly enough for you. If not, let it ferment longer.

Once the kombucha suits your taste, transfer the bottle to the refrigerator.

Storage note: This kombucha will last in the sealed container in the fridge for 1 year but will turn to vinegar over time. It is still fine to drink but might be better used as vinegar because of the sour taste. Once open, the carbonation will start to decrease—just as with regular store-bought soda.

STRAWBERRY KOMBUCHA MARGARITA

My husband and I went to Mexico for our 30th anniversary and attended a salsa and margarita class. This strawberry margarita was inspired by a recipe we made there, and it's become my afternoon pick-me-up. I love it because it's tasty and brings back such good memories.

Makes 1 serving

¼ cup fresh-squeezed lime juice

1½ teaspoons Celtic Sea Salt

½ cup Basic Kombucha (page 62)

1 cup strawberries, hulled

2 cups ice

A few drops stevia or a drizzle of honey

Place the lime juice on a small plate and the salt on another.

Dip the rim of a glass in the lime juice and then the salt.

Place the remaining lime juice in the blender along with the kombucha, strawberries, ice, and stevia. Blend until well combined, then serve in the salt-rimmed glass.

GRAPE KOMBUCHA WITH COCONUT WHIPPED CREAM

This drink, which is made with frozen grapes and the cream from coconut milk, is a fun way to have kombucha. And it's great for the summer—nice and refreshing.

Makes 1 serving

½ cup frozen grapes

1 cup Second-Fermented Kombucha, using grape juice (page 64)

¼ cup Coconut Whipped Cream (page 179)

....

Place frozen grapes in a tall glass and pour the kombucha over the top.

Top with Coconut Whipped Cream and serve immediately.

CANDY CANE KOMBUCHA

My daughter Maci made this for Christmastime and I loved it so much that I couldn't stop drinking it. And I wasn't the only one: the proprietors of a vegan raw food restaurant called Café Gratitude heard about it and asked if they could use this recipe on their menu. We were so excited! Café Gratitude is one of my favorite restaurants and one of the few around Kansas City that have kombucha, kefir, and cultured veggies on their menus.

Makes 3 quarts; six 16-ounce servings

12 cups Basic Kombucha (page 62)

3 organic candy canes

....

Fill 6 bottles with kombucha and place half a candy cane in each.

Seal the bottles and let the kombucha sit on your kitchen counter, out of direct sunlight, for 3 days to 2 weeks. The fermentation time will depend on how sweet your kombucha was to start with and the temperature in your house.

Check the bottles often in order to taste the kombucha and to release the pressure. When the kombucha is bubbly, it is done.

Place the bottles in the refrigerator.

Storage note: This kombucha will last in sealed containers in the fridge for a year but will turn to vinegar over time. It is still fine to drink but might be better used as vinegar because of the sour taste. Once open, the carbonation will start to decrease—just as with regular store-bought soda.

FENNEL KOMBUCHA

Adding fennel juice to kombucha makes it taste like licorice—something I love. And using freshly extracted fennel juice makes your kombucha faster fermenting and bubblier because fresh juice has higher levels of enzymes. Enjoy this healing and slightly licorice-y drink!

A note before you begin: This recipe requires a juicer.

Makes 16 ounces; 1 serving

¼ bulb fennel

1⅞ cups Basic Kombucha (page 62)

Juice the fennel, and then add the fennel juice and kombucha to a sturdy bottle.

Clamp the cap closed and date the bottle so you know when the second fermentation began.

Let the kombucha sit on your kitchen counter, out of direct sunlight, for 5 to 7 days.

Check the kombucha after each week to see if it is bubbly enough for you. If not, let it ferment longer.

Once the kombucha suits your taste, transfer the bottle to the refrigerator.

Storage note: This kombucha will last in the sealed container in the fridge for 1 year but will turn to vinegar over time. It is still fine to drink but might be better used as vinegar because of the sour taste. Once open, the carbonation will start to decrease—just as with regular store-bought soda.

CHAPTER 13

Condiments, Dressings, Flavorings, and Pickles

COCONUT WHIPPED CREAM

This discovery I made is super delicious—and it adds just a bit of variety when you're making anything that uses whipped cream. Two brands of coconut milk I recommend for this are Thai Kitchen and Whole Foods 365 Everyday Value organic coconut milk. If you add a teaspoon of EcoBloom, you will make this a prebiotic and feed your good bacteria, too.

Makes 12 servings

1 can coconut milk

1 teaspoon EcoBloom (optional)

Place the can of coconut milk in the fridge and leave it for a few hours.

Remove the can from the fridge, making sure not to shake it. You want the cream to stay separated.

Open the can and spoon the cream off the top, leaving the coconut water.

Place the cream and the EcoBloom (if using) in a small bowl and beat, using an electric mixer, until it's light and fluffy.

Storage note: This whipped cream will harden and set in the fridge over time. It will keep for 1 to 2 weeks in a sealed container in the fridge.

KOMBUCHA STRAWBERRY MAPLE SYRUP

This is a wonderful topping for pancakes and waffles or even a bowl of fruit or oatmeal. Remember that kombucha has good yeasts in it that cannot be killed by heat, so even if your pancakes are piping hot, you'll still get probiotics in this topping.

Makes 1 pint; 32 1-tablespoon servings

1½ cups strawberries, hulled

2 tablespoons chia seeds

2 tablespoons maple syrup

2 tablespoons Basic Kombucha (page 62)

Place all the ingredients in a blender and process until smooth.

FERMENTED GARLIC

This recipe is one of my daughter Maci's creations. She made it for her brother, who loved it and begged her for more. Fermented garlic becomes super bubbly when it cultures. You will see lots of bubbles in the jar. It can be used in any recipe that calls for garlic—and it'll give the dish an extra-special little zing.

Makes 1 cup; 16 1-tablespoon servings

⅛ teaspoon Cutting Edge Starter Culture plus ¼ cup water, or 2 tablespoons Kefir Whey (page 57)

¾ cup garlic cloves, peeled

½ teaspoon Celtic Sea Salt

If using the starter culture, stir together the culture and water. Let the mixture sit while you prepare the other ingredients—around 10 minutes.

Place the garlic and salt in a 1-pint glass or ceramic container that can be securely sealed.

Add the starter culture or the whey and fill the jar with filtered water, leaving 1 inch of headspace to let the garlic bubble and expand as it ferments.

Seal the container and let it sit on your kitchen counter, out of direct sunlight, for 3 to 4 days.

Check the garlic every day to make sure it is fully submerged. If it has risen above the water, simply push it down so it is fully covered again. If white spots of yeast have formed on any unsubmerged garlic, do not worry. Remember, this isn't harmful. Just scoop out the yeast and garlic it's on and push the rest back under the water. (See FAQs on page 69 for more information.)

When the garlic is done fermenting, place it in the refrigerator.

Storage note: This garlic can be stored in an airtight container in the refrigerator for up to 9 months.

KOMBUCHA MAYONNAISE

This is the only mayo I use. The taste is delicious, and there are no chemicals or preservatives; store-bought mayo can't compete. This mayo is so easy to make—it takes only about four minutes and uses just a few ingredients—that you can whip it up whenever you need it.

A note before you begin: This recipe calls for consuming raw eggs, and people with compromised immune systems should not do so. For those of you who do choose to make the mayo, I recommend using the freshest eggs possible. The best choice is to get eggs directly from a farm or a reliable vendor at a farmers' market, but eggs from cage-free, pasture-raised chickens, which are sold in most grocery stores, are also generally safe.

Makes 2 cups; 32 1-tablespoon servings

¼ cup Basic Kombucha (page 62)

2 large egg yolks

½ teaspoon mustard powder

½ teaspoon onion powder

½ teaspoon garlic powder

½ teaspoon Celtic Sea Salt

1 cup extra-virgin olive oil

Place the kombucha, egg yolks, mustard powder, onion powder, garlic powder, and salt in the work bowl of a food processor and pulse until mixed.

With the food processor running, slowly drizzle the olive oil through the feed tube.

Process for 4 to 5 minutes until the mixture thickens and is the creamy consistency of store-bought mayo.

Storage note: This mayonnaise can be stored in a sealed airtight container in the refrigerator for up to 3 months.

LEMON KEFIR LABNEH

Labneh is a soft cream cheese made from strained yogurt or kefir. I make mine with lemon because it pairs so well with so many things. You'll notice it in a number of recipes throughout the book. What's more, lemons are great detoxifiers, immune builders, and prebiotics.

Makes 2 servings

½ cup Kefir Cheese (page 57)

1 tablespoon lemon juice

1 tablespoon lemon zest

1 tablespoon honey

Mix all the ingredients in a small bowl until well combined.

FERMENTED FRUIT JAM

My grandma lived on an island in Nova Scotia, and she made the best raspberry jam in the whole world. She had raspberry bushes in her backyard, and the raspberries would get really fat from the saltwater air that they grew in. I tried to create their unique flavor with this recipe so I can remember my summer days in Nova Scotia.

Makes 2 1/2 cups; 40 1-tablespoon servings

2 cups fresh raspberries

2 tablespoons honey

2 tablespoons chia seeds

2 tablespoons Peach Kombucha Sangria (page 167)

1 teaspoon vanilla

....

Place all the ingredients in a blender or food processor and pulse until the jam has a texture you like.

Transfer the mixture to a container with a lid and allow it to set in the fridge for at least an hour.

Storage note: The jam will keep in a covered jar in the refrigerator for 5 days.

KEFIR RANCH DRESSING

My husband loves ranch dressing, but I hate the commercial stuff. Most of it is full of MSG and artificial ingredients. So I spent a long time trying to create the perfect ranch dressing for him. He's finicky, so when he liked this, I knew I'd hit the jackpot.

A note before you begin: In the ingredients below, I've listed a range for the amount of kefir to use. The only thing this changes is the thickness of the dressing. If you like a thick ranch, use less kefir. If you want a thin dressing, use more.

Makes 1¾ cups; 28 1-tablespoon servings

½ cup Kombucha Mayonnaise (page 182)

½ cup Kefir Cheese (page 57)

¼ to ½ cup Basic Kefir (page 51),

⅛ cup chopped flat-leaf parsley

1 large clove garlic, quartered

1 teaspoon white wine vinegar

1 teaspoon Worcestershire sauce

1 teaspoon Bragg Organic Sea Kelp Delight Seasoning

1 teaspoon onion salt or dehydrated minced onion

½ teaspoon paprika

½ teaspoon freshly ground black pepper

⅛ teaspoon cayenne pepper

Mix together all the ingredients in a food processor or blender on high speed until the mixture is smooth and creamy.

Transfer the dressing to a covered container and chill in the refrigerator for at least 1 hour to let the flavors meld.

Storage note: This dressing can be stored in an airtight container in the refrigerator for up to 1 month.

CULTURED GREEN TOMATO RELISH

My daughter Maci got married this year and moved to a farm with her husband, which has given her time to try all sorts of new recipes. She adapted this one from the sweet pickle relish in my last book. Luckily for her, her new husband likes fermenting. It's cute to see pictures of them fermenting together. It makes me very happy!

Makes 1 quart; 16 ¼-cup servings

⅛ teaspoon Cutting Edge Starter Culture plus ¼ cup water, or 2 tablespoons Kefir Whey (page 57)

3 cups chopped fresh green tomatoes

½ cup diced onions

¼ cup honey or maple syrup

½ red pepper, seeded and diced

1½ teaspoons Celtic Sea Salt

1 tablespoon whole celery seeds

1 teaspoon turmeric

½ tablespoon yellow mustard seeds

....

If using the starter culture, stir together the culture and water. Let the mixture sit while you prepare the other ingredients—around 10 minutes.

Place the remaining ingredients in a food processor and pulse until well combined and the mixture has a relish consistency.

Add the starter culture or kefir whey to the food processor and pulse again two or three times to combine.

Transfer the mixture into a canning jar and fill the jar with filtered water, leaving 2 to 3 inches of headspace to let the relish bubble and expand as it ferments.

Seal the container and let it sit on your kitchen counter, out of direct sunlight, for 3 days.

Check the relish every day to make sure it is fully submerged. If it has risen above the water, simply push it down so it is fully covered again. If white spots of yeast have formed on any unsubmerged relish, do not worry. Remember, this isn't harmful. Just scoop out the yeast and relish it's on and push the rest back under the water. (See FAQs on page 69 for more information.)

When the relish is done fermenting, place it in the refrigerator.

Storage note: This relish can be kept in an airtight jar in the refrigerator for up to 1 year.

SWEET FERMENTED PICKLE RELISH

One time, I made this pickle relish, stuck it in the back of the fridge, and forgot about it. A year later I found it and opened it. It was bubbly and tasted really, really good. The added honey makes this recipe unique, and it ferments like a fine wine.

Makes 1 quart; 32 2-tablespoon servings

¼ teaspoon Cutting Edge Starter Culture plus ½ cup water, or ¼ cup Kefir Whey (page 57)

3 small cucumbers

½ onion

½ red bell pepper

½ cup honey or maple syrup

1½ tablespoons Celtic Sea Salt

1 tablespoon whole celery seeds

1½ teaspoons yellow mustard seeds

1 teaspoon turmeric

....

If using the starter culture, stir together the culture and water. Let the mixture sit while you prepare the other ingredients—around 10 minutes. If using kefir whey, add it when the recipe calls for culture.

Chop the cucumbers and onion and mix them together in a large bowl.

Transfer the mixture into a 1-quart glass or ceramic container that can be securely sealed.

Press the veggies down lightly with a spoon to pack them.

Seed and dice the red pepper.

Combine the culture, bell pepper, honey, salt, celery seeds, mustard seeds, and turmeric and pour the mixture over the vegetables.

Add filtered water to cover, leaving 1 inch of headspace to let the vegetables bubble and expand as they ferment.

Seal the container and let it sit on your kitchen counter, out of direct sunlight, for 3 days.

Check the relish every day to make sure it is fully submerged. If it has risen above the water, simply push it down so it is fully covered again. If white spots of yeast have formed on any unsubmerged relish, do not worry. Remember, this isn't harmful. Just scoop out the yeast and relish it's on and push the rest back under the water. (See FAQs on page 69 for more information.)

When the relish is done fermenting, place it in the refrigerator.

Storage note: This relish can be kept in an airtight container in the refrigerator for up to 3 weeks.

BILLION BIOTICLAND DRESSING

This tastes just like Thousand Island dressing. I just changed the name to suit me—and the billions of probiotics that reside within it.

Makes ¾ cup; 12 1-tablespoon servings

½ cup Kombucha Mayonnaise (page 182)

2 tablespoons Probiotic Ketchup (page 189)

1 tablespoon Basic Kombucha (page 62)

2 teaspoons honey

2 teaspoons Sweet Fermented Pickle Relish (page 187)

1 teaspoon finely minced white onion

⅛ teaspoon salt

Combine all ingredients in a small bowl and stir well to combine. Refrigerate for at least 2 hours before using.

PROBIOTIC KETCHUP

So many people love ketchup, but the store-bought variety has a lot of sugar in it. I was looking for a way to reduce the amount of sugar in ketchup and came up with this. My ketchup is super-easy to make and has a lot less sugar—and it's filled with probiotics!

Makes 4 cups; 64 1-tablespoon servings

3 cups tomato paste, preferably organic

½ cup maple syrup

½ cup Asian fish sauce

¼ teaspoon Cutting Edge Starter Culture or ¼ cup Kefir Whey (page 57)

3 cloves garlic, peeled and mashed

1 tablespoon Celtic Sea Salt

½ teaspoon ground cumin

¼ teaspoon ground cinnamon

¼ teaspoon cayenne pepper

Put all the ingredients into a large bowl and stir together until combined.

Pour the mixture into two 1-pint jars or one 1-quart jar, leaving approximately 1 inch of headspace to let the ketchup ferment.

Seal the jar(s), and leave on the kitchen counter, out of direct sunlight, for 2 days; then transfer the ketchup to the refrigerator.

Storage note: This ketchup can be stored in the sealed jar(s) in the refrigerator for up to 3 months.

APPLE KEFIR DRESSING

This is the dressing for Salad in a Fermenting Jar (page 144), which I take everywhere since it travels well. This is also my sister's favorite dressing, and I know why: it has the flavor of ranch dressing with just a slight hint of apple.

Makes ¾ cup; 12 1-tablespoon servings

½ cup Kefir Cheese (page 57)

2 teaspoons garlic powder

2 teaspoons onion powder

2 tablespoons Basic Kombucha (page 62)

2 tablespoons apple juice

1½ teaspoons honey

. . . .

Place all the ingredients in a small bowl and whisk until smooth.

Storage note: This dressing can be stored in a sealed jar in the refrigerator for up to 3 weeks.

CURRIED APPLE RELISH

I love to serve this along with a plate of fruit, cheese, and crackers because it adds just a little extra kick. It is especially nice with a good Brie. Mmm . . .

Makes 1 quart; 48 4-teaspoon servings

⅛ teaspoon Cutting Edge Starter Culture plus ¼ cup water, or 2 tablespoons Kefir Whey (page 57)

½ apple, preferably green

2 medium cucumbers

½ cup raisins

½ onion

1 clove garlic

⅛ cup Sucanat

1 teaspoon sweet curry powder

1 teaspoon Celtic Sea Salt

½ teaspoon ground ginger

⅛ teaspoon ground cloves

⅛ teaspoon cinnamon

....

If using the starter culture, stir together the culture and water. Let the mixture sit while you prepare the other ingredients—around 10 minutes. If using kefir whey, add it when the recipe calls for culture.

Core the apple and cut it into chunks. Cut the cucumbers into chunks. Then place the apple, cucumber, raisins, onion, and garlic in a food processor and pulse until the mixture is the consistency of relish.

Place the mixture in a canning jar and add the Sucanat and the spices.

Add the culture or kefir whey. Add filtered water to cover, leaving 2 inches of headspace to let the vegetables bubble and expand as they ferment.

Seal the container and let it sit on your kitchen counter, out of direct sunlight, for 2 days.

Check the relish every day to make sure it is fully submerged. If it has risen above the water, simply push it down so it is fully covered again. If white spots of yeast have formed on any unsubmerged relish, do not worry. Remember, this isn't harmful. Just scoop out the yeast and relish it's on and push the rest back under the water. (See FAQs on page 69 for more information.)

When the relish is done fermenting, place it in the refrigerator.

Storage note: This relish can be kept in an airtight jar in the refrigerator for up to 9 months.

AFTERWORD: LOVING YOUR HUNDRED TRILLION FRIENDS

I hope you will enjoy your exploration of the world of cultured foods. I hope it will bless you and teach you how you are supposed to live your life: healthy, happy, and spreading joy to others. After I incorporated these foods into my life they began to change me from the inside out, and now I can't go back. Without them my aliments return, and I never want to feel like that again. Feeling the best you can is addictive! You stop worrying about sickness and disease, and you begin to believe that your body will take care of you on this journey called life.

So be good to yourself and take life at your own pace. As you begin to add these foods to your diet, you will come to look at harmful foods with disdain and you'll desire healthier foods like never before. This is how it was always meant to be. You and your hundred trillion friends are an unbeatable combination. Feed them what they need and they will take care of you. Just you wait and see!

— **Donna**

APPENDIX:
YOUR 21-DAY TRILOGY PROGRAM

Many people I work with mistakenly think I eat only cultured foods. Sure, some days are pretty heavy on the cultured-food front, but for the most part, I simply look to incorporate small quantities of the Trilogy into my daily life. On a typical day, I have a kefir smoothie for breakfast, 8 to 16 ounces of kombucha throughout the day, and a scoop or two of cultured veggies with lunch and dinner. The rest of my food centers on a lot of fresh fruits and vegetables, which provide me with excellent prebiotics. We're not talking huge amounts of any single part of the Trilogy.

Eating healthy should be easy. As I said before, I don't create hard recipes, because I want people to actually make them. I won't hassle with complicated instructions, so why would I expect you to? In that same line of thinking, I have created here what I think is a super-simple way to get the Trilogy into your life. It walks you step-by-step through buying, prepping, and eating kefir, kombucha, and cultured vegetables.

A note before you begin: This program introduces all parts of the Trilogy to you over the course of 21 days. Depending on your health, you could experience a Herxheimer reaction (see page 44). If you aren't feeling well after consuming this many probiotic foods, you have a couple of choices. You can slow down—put a day or two between each day's instructions in the program—or you can power through. This is a serious amount of bacteria, and it will clean you out! But if you can't handle the symptoms, don't try to force your way through it. Eating cultured foods is about feeling good.

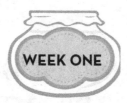

Day 1: Shop for Kefir Materials and Other Foodstuffs

In this program, you will be shopping for materials one day each week, but this first shopping trip is going to be the biggest. Today you will gather the materials necessary to make kefir and kefir cheese. You will also get the perishable food items needed for the week **and** the nonperishable items that will be used throughout the program.

Before you go shopping, there is one decision you need to make: Will you use kefir grains or kefir packets? In making this choice, there are a few things to consider. Ask yourself these two questions:

Question 1: Do you want to make dairy kefir or nondairy kefir? If you want to make dairy kefir, either method will work. If you want to make nondairy kefir, you should use the grains.

Question 2: If you want to make dairy kefir, do you want a stronger kefir that takes a bit more work, or a kefir that packs less punch but is easier to make? In this program, if you use the packets, you will make kefir once a week and there is no storing or caring for grains; however, the kefir won't be quite as powerful. If you use the grains, the kefir will have more strains of healthy bacteria, but you will need to make it four days each week of the program and store it the other three.

Once you've made this decision, grab the shopping lists below and get started:

Basic/Kefir Cheese Materials:

- *Starter culture:* You can use Easy Kefir or kefir grains. If you know somebody who has grains to share, get those. Or you can acquire these items online. I offer them in my store (www.culturedfoodlife.com/store), or you can get them from Wise Choice Market (www.wisechoicemarket.com). Just remember, if you plan to make kefir with nondairy milk, kefir grains are the preferred method. (If you are ordering from my site, you may want to check out the materials listed on days 7 and 14 also—then you can order everything at once.)

- *Two 1-quart canning jars:* You will need two glass jars with lids. Plastic lids are better, but metal will work, too.

- *Strainer:* Many people say that you must use a plastic strainer to strain the grains from kefir, but I have found that stainless steel and plastic both work. So if you're using grains, choose what works best for you. For making kefir cheese, I've found that a stainless steel strainer works best.

- *Coffee filters:* Your standard 8-cup, auto-drip coffee filters will work fine.

- *Deep bowl:* You want a bowl on which you can balance your strainer when making kefir cheese. Make sure the bowl is deep enough to collect the whey that separates from the cheese.

- *4 cups of milk:* Almost any type of milk is acceptable. For dairy milk, raw, whole, reduced fat, nonfat, pasteurized, homogenized—it all works. For nondairy milks, coconut, almond, and cashew work very well and are available in most stores. They're also pretty easy to make if you want to do that. You can find a great recipe from wellness warrior and best-selling author Kris Carr at kriscarr.com/recipe/basic-nutseed-milk.

Other Foodstuffs:

- Black pepper
- Celtic Sea Salt
- Cinnamon
- Cocoa powder
- Coriander
- Liquid stevia
- Oatmeal (old-fashioned or rolled oats will work)
- Pumpkin pie spice

- Shredded coconut
- Stevia or maple syrup
- Vanilla extract
- Chia seeds
- ¼ cup chopped pecans
- Sliced almonds
- 1½ cups fresh or frozen blueberries
- ½ cup frozen or fresh mixed berries
- 1 quart unsweetened almond milk (this will make recipes in weeks 1 and 2)

Day 2: Make Kefir!

Over the course of this 21-day program, you will make more than 10 cups of kefir. As you know, there are two ways to make kefir—using packets and using grains.

- If you are using Easy Kefir packets, you will make 4 cups at a time—4 today, 4 on day 8, and 4 on day 14.
- If you are using kefir grains, you will make 1 cup each day for 4 days in a row, and then you will store the grains for 3 days before beginning again.

Don't worry—I'll remind you what to do each day! So today, make either 4 cups, using packets (see page 52 for step-by-step instructions) or 1 cup, using grains (see page 53 for step-by-step instructions).

Day 3: Be Proud! You Made Kefir!

All right, let's take a look at and taste your kefir to make sure it came out right. Is it slightly thick, like drinkable yogurt? Is it tart and sour? If you answered yes to both of these questions, you've successfully made kefir. Congratulations! If your kefir is not tart or sour and still looks and tastes like milk, then let it ferment longer.

Once your kefir is properly fermented, it's ready to drink. However, if you used grains, you'll need to separate them from the kefir using a strainer.

While I'd love to say that you should drink as much of this kefir as you want, please don't do that unless you make more to replace it. I've incorporated all the kefir you've just made into recipes in this program, so drinking it now will mean that you'll be short in the future.

What if? If your kefir separated into clear whey and curds, don't worry. This isn't bad; it simply means your kefir is overfermented. Either the ratio of grains to milk was too high, or your house was on the warmer side. Either of these will make your kefir ferment faster. It is still fine to drink. Just remove the grains (if you used them) and then shake up the kefir. I have a great video on my site that shows exactly what has happened. The site also offers other tips on how to make it creamy again:

- www.culturedfoodlife.com/the-trilogy/kefir/kefir-separating
- www.culturedfoodlife.com/the-trilogy/kefir/how-to-make-your-kefir-creamy -again

If you're making kefir using grains, make another cup of kefir today.

Day 4: Enjoy Your Kefir for Breakfast

Try out the Coco-Nutty Berry Kefir (page 76) for breakfast. It's a great entry into using kefir in recipes because it's easy and utterly delicious.

If you're making kefir using grains, make another cup of kefir today.

Day 5: Prep Your Breakfast

Today you won't eat any part of the Trilogy—just let your system recover from your first dose of kefir. But before you head to bed, prepare some Overnight Blueberry Kefir Oatmeal (page 85). It'll make a nice treat for you in the morning.

If you're making kefir using grains, make another cup of kefir today.

Day 6: Eat Your Blueberry Kefir Oatmeal

It's another easy day today, folks. Just eat that delicious breakfast you made last night.

If you're making kefir using grains, prep the grains for storage today. See page 54 for instructions on how to do this. You will make kefir again on Day 9.

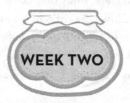

WEEK TWO

Day 7: Shop for Cultured Veggie Materials and Other Foodstuffs, Make Kefir Cheese and Whey, and Prep Pudding

It's your second shopping day! Today you will buy the items needed to make cultured veggies—in this instance, Lemon Kraut—along with the perishable items for the recipes this week. Here are your lists:

Cultured Veggie/Lemon Kraut Materials:

- *Starter culture:* I recommend that you make the Lemon Kraut by using Cutting Edge Starter Culture, which you can buy in the store on my site: www.culturedfoodlife.com/store. However, you can also make this by using the kefir whey you will make today.

- *Two 1-quart canning jars or one ½-gallon jar:* You will need one or two glass jars with lids. Plastic lids are better but metal will work, too.

- 1 small head cabbage (about 1 pound)

- 1 apple

- 1 lemon (3 total; see shopping list below)

Other Foodstuffs:

- 1 avocado
- 4 fresh basil leaves
- 2 lemons
- 2 oranges

You will also need to make four more cups of kefir this week, so pick up more milk if you need it.

Today is also the day you're going to make some kefir cheese. It may seem that I'm telling you to do a lot of things today, but really, making kefir cheese is so easy that it's not really even a task. I make kefir cheese several times a week. It's a cross between sour cream and cream cheese and can be used in any recipe that calls for one of those ingredients. It's easy to do: just prep it tonight, and then you'll have fresh cheese and whey tomorrow. Here is what you will need:

- Stainless steel strainer
- Deep bowl to place the strainer in
- Coffee filter
- 2 cups kefir

Once you have these materials in hand, see page 57 for step-by-step instructions on how to make kefir cheese and whey.

And before you go to bed, whip up some Overnight Kefir Brownie Pudding (page 157) for tomorrow.

Day 8: Make Lemon Kraut—and Treat Yourself

Today is the day you will make Lemon Kraut. See page 124 for instructions.

Once you're done, treat yourself with that brownie pudding you made last night! You deserve it!

If you're making kefir using starter culture packets, make 4 cups of kefir today. See page 52 for instructions.

Day 9: Use Your Kefir Cheese

You're not going to see any results for the cultured veggies for a couple of days, but do check on them to make sure they are fully submerged in water and free of kahm yeast. If they have risen to the top, open the jar and push them under the water. If there is yeast growing, remove the yeast and the veggies it is on.

For lunch today, enjoy your kefir cheese in Kefir Orange Cups (page 95).

If you're making kefir using grains, take them out of storage and make a cup of kefir today. See page 53 for instructions.

Day 10: Drink Your Kefir

Kefir smoothies are such an easy and filling breakfast, which is why I drink them all the time. However, you can also have them for a midafternoon snack—or anytime you need a pick-me-up. Try the Sun-Fresh Smoothie (page 82) today.

Also remember to check your veggies to make sure they are fully submerged in water and free of kahm yeast. If they have risen to the top, open the jar and push them under the water. If there is yeast growing, remove the yeast and the veggies it is on.

If you're making kefir using grains, make another cup of kefir today.

Day 11: Second-Ferment Your Kefir

This is the way I make all of my kefir. I add a small piece of fruit or fruit peel to my already-made kefir and let it ferment for an hour or even up to a day on the counter. It increases the B vitamins and also changes the flavor, making it less sour and much more delicious. I highly recommend it. See step-by-step instructions on how to second-ferment kefir (using lemon) on page 56. Today you will make only half a batch of second-fermented kefir. So you will use only 1 cup of your prepared kefir.

Also remember to check your veggies to make sure they are fully submerged in water and free of kahm yeast. If they have risen to the top, open the jar and push them under the water. If there is yeast growing, remove the yeast and the veggies it is on.

If you're making kefir using grains, make another cup of kefir today.

Day 12: Check Your Veggies and Have a Cup of Second-Fermented Kefir

This is the fifth day in your veggies' fermentation, so they may be ready to eat. Or they should at least be well on their way. Let's check on their progress. You should start to see bubbles in your jar; however, you might not see these if you didn't use a culture or your house is on the cold side. The water should also be getting cloudy. This is a great sign that your vegetables are fermenting and making a probiotic-rich brine. If your veggies are not bubbly or cloudy, your home might be on the colder end of the spectrum, which means that you just need to wait a little longer.

Celebrate your success by drinking some of your second-fermented kefir! Have as much or as little of it as you'd like. We won't be using it in any other recipes.

If you're making kefir using grains, make another cup of kefir today.

Day 13: Try Your Lemon Kraut and Make some Kefir Cheese

Your Lemon Kraut should be done about now, so I want you to taste it. See if it tastes sour, like sauerkraut. If yes, have a spoonful! Then place the jar in the fridge. The kraut will continue to ferment slowly and will get more intensely flavored over time. If the kraut didn't taste sour, leave it to ferment for another day or two.

Today you will also need to make another batch of kefir cheese and whey. See page 57 for step-by-step instructions.

If you're making kefir using grains, you'll prep them for storage today. See page 54 for instructions on how to do this. You will make kefir again on day 16.

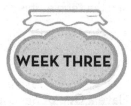

WEEK THREE

Day 14: Shop for Kombucha Materials and Other Foodstuffs—and Eat Some Kraut

Here we are at your final shopping day! Today you will buy the items needed to make kombucha, along with the perishable items for the recipes this week. Here are your lists:

Kombucha Materials:

- *Kombucha starter kit:* To make kombucha, you need a kombucha SCOBY and 1 cup of already-made kombucha tea. If you know somebody who makes kombucha, you can likely get these things from her—she'll probably be excited that someone wants to take a SCOBY off her hands! If you don't know anyone who does this, you can always order it from the store on my site: www.culturedfoodlife.com/store.

- *Container:* You will need a 1-gallon jar or lead-free crock.

- *Linen or cloth napkin:* This needs to be big enough to fit completely over the top of the jar or crock you've selected.

- *Rubber band:* Make sure this is big enough to go around the neck of the jug or crock you've selected. This will hold the napkin in place.

- *Six 16-ounce glass bottles:* Make sure these are good, sturdy bottles with clamp-down lids. You can repurpose beer bottles such as those from Grolsch, or you can buy new thick-glass bottles that are specifically designed for brewing. Bottles bought at craft stores aren't as sturdy and may explode.

- *Brew belt:* This gadget is optional but highly recommended. It is basically a plug-in heater for your jar or crock. You wrap it around the container you're using to brew your kombucha, and it keeps the tea at a consistent temperature between 75°F and 80°F.

- 1 cup sugar (Sucanat, white sugar, or coconut sugar)
- 4 or 5 tea bags; you can use black or green tea, and organic is best
- 3 quarts filtered water (not distilled)

Other Foodstuffs:

- 1 avocado
- 3 bananas
- 2 tablespoons fresh chopped cilantro
- 2-inch piece fresh ginger
- 1 lemon
- 1 lime
- 1 tablespoon finely chopped fresh rosemary
- 1 large russet potato or sweet potato
- 1½ cups chopped strawberries
- ½ cup shredded or grated Parmesan cheese
- 1½ tablespoons toasted sesame seeds
- 1 quart unsweetened almond milk
- 1 teaspoon loose-leaf chai tea or the contents of 1 chai tea bag
- 3 tablespoons pumpkin puree
- 1 egg

You will also need to make 4 more cups of kefir to use this week, so pick up more milk if you need it.

Have a couple spoonfuls of Lemon Kraut today with your lunch or dinner. It'll make your belly happy!

If you're making kefir using starter culture packets, make 4 cups of kefir today. See page 52 for instructions.

Day 15: Make Your Kombucha and Have an Avocado Boat

We're finally making that final piece of the Trilogy: kombucha. Check out page 62 for step-by-step instructions. You can see photos of the kombucha-making process at www.culturedfoodlife .com/the-trilogy/kombucha/how-to-make-kombucha.

Today you can also have one of my favorite dishes for lunch: the Cultured Avocado Boat (page 109).

Day 16: Eat Cultured Veggies and Kefir—Together!

You are not going to see anything for a couple of days with your kombucha, so we'll hold off on checking it for a little while. But in the meantime, enjoy a combo of your kefir cheese and Lemon Kraut. Make some Parmesan Crisps and Kraut (page 96) and have it for a snack.

Oh, yeah—and throw three bananas in the freezer tonight before you go to bed. You'll need them on day 17 and day 19. Remember to peel and chop them first!

If you're making kefir using grains, take them out of storage and make a cup of kefir today. See page 53 for instructions.

Day 17: Relax with Some Delicious Kefir Ice Cream

Today simply sit back and enjoy the probiotic benefits of some Superfast Banana Kefir Ice Cream (page 160).

If you're making kefir using grains, make another cup of kefir today.

Day 18: Check your Kombucha, Make Kefir Cheese, and Eat Your Veggies

Let's start today by checking on your kombucha. A clear film, white dots, or a thick disc should be forming on the surface of your kombucha. This is your new SCOBY. The kombucha should also look cloudy at this point.

If a new SCOBY isn't forming and the kombucha is still clear, it's likely because your home is colder than the optimum fermenting temperature, which is about 80°F. My suggestion is to use a brew belt to regulate the temperature, or place your jar or crock on a heating pad on low heat, or make your home a bit warmer. Or you can simply let the kombucha ferment longer. It will ferment at a cooler temperature, but it will take longer.

When you make kombucha, the tea will change in appearance as a result of fermentation. The active yeast and bacteria will eat the sugars out of the tea and make those sugars into probiotics for you. Check out step-by-step pictures of kombucha fermenting at www.cultured foodlife.com/the-trilogy/kombucha/how-to-make-kombucha.

What if? If the SCOBY you used to start your kombucha has sunk to the bottom of the jar or crock, this is completely fine.

What if? If you see stringy things hanging from the SCOBY or spots on it, do not worry. It may look scary, but this is just the good yeast that makes probiotics and carbonation in your brew.

Today you will also make half of the standard Kefir Cheese recipe. So you will use only 1 cup of kefir. See page 57 for step-by-step instructions.

Also make sure to eat a couple of spoonfuls of Lemon Kraut today with your lunch or dinner. Keep those probiotics coming!

If you're making kefir using grains, make another cup of kefir today.

Day 19: Mix Up some Kefir Cheese and Veggies and Prep some Breakfast

I make the recipe Veggies Love Kefir Cheese multiple times each week. It's so good and so easy. So whip up some for yourself. The recipe is on page 99, and while it calls for Orangeade Kraut, for now you can simply make it with your Lemon Kraut. It's just as delicious.

And before you go to bed, prep an Overnight Strawberry Kefir Pudding (page 86). It'll be a delightful treat when you wake up.

If you're making kefir using grains, you'll prep them for storage today. See page 54 for instructions on how to do this. You will make kefir again on . . . whatever day you want. You don't have to make it again for this program!

Day 20: Test Your Kombucha and Second-Ferment It, Then Drink Some Chai

Start your day out with that delicious strawberry pudding you made. Then check your kombucha.

It has been six days since you started making your kombucha, which means that it could be ready. So go ahead and taste it. Pour off a couple of ounces of tea and drink it. If it tastes sweet, then not all the sugar has been converted to probiotics, so it's not quite ready. But if it tastes like a tart, sparkling apple cider, it's ready! You can now transfer it into bottles and place it in the fridge. Don't forget to save a cup of tea to make your next batch of kombucha.

If your kombucha is ready, let's second-ferment some of it. While you can do this by using any kind of 100 percent fruit juice, let's instead make one of my most popular recipes: Ginger Kombucha (page 170).

Blend up the Chai Kefir Smoothie (page 71) today whenever you want a treat. This is one of my favorites! It's so decadent.

Day 21: Consume the Whole Trilogy

Well, folks, you've made it to the end of the program. So for this last day, let's have all three pieces of the Trilogy. It's pretty simple. Just have a Cultured Baked Potato (page 112) for lunch, along with ½ cup of kombucha. In this one meal you will consume tons of probiotics!

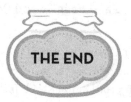

THE END

I hope this simple program has helped you understand how easy it is to make and eat cultured foods. You just have to make a few and include them in and with your meals. There are a lot more recipes to try, and the more you make them and have them on hand, the more you will eat and drink them. And soon you'll discover that you have transformed your kitchen and the universe inside of you—along with your health!

METRIC CONVERSION TABLES

STANDARD CUP	FINE POWDER (E.G., FLOUR)	GRAIN (E.G., RICE)	GRANULAR (E.G., SUGAR)	LIQUID SOLIDS (E.G., BUTTER)	LIQUID (E.G., MILK)
1	140 g	150 g	190 g	200 g	240 ml
¾	105 g	113 g	143 g	150 g	180 ml
⅔	93 g	100 g	125 g	133 g	160 ml
½	70 g	75 g	95 g	100 g	120 ml
⅓	47 g	50 g	63 g	67 g	80 ml
¼	35 g	38 g	48 g	50 g	60 ml
⅛	18 g	19 g	24 g	25 g	30 ml

USEFUL EQUIVALENTS FOR LIQUID INGREDIENTS BY VOLUME

¼ tsp				1 ml	
½ tsp				2 ml	
1 tsp				5 ml	
3 tsp	1 tbsp		½ fl oz	15 ml	
	2 tbsp	⅛ cup	1 fl oz	30 ml	
	4 tbsp	¼ cup	2 fl oz	60 ml	
	5⅓ tbsp	⅓ cup	3 fl oz	80 ml	
	8 tbsp	½ cup	4 fl oz	120 ml	
	10⅔ tbsp	⅔ cup	5 fl oz	160 ml	
	12 tbsp	¾ cup	6 fl oz	180 ml	
	16 tbsp	1 cup	8 fl oz	240 ml	
	1 pt	2 cups	16 fl oz	480 ml	
	1 qt	4 cups	32 fl oz	960 ml	
			33 fl oz	1000 ml	1 l

USEFUL EQUIVALENTS FOR DRY INGREDIENTS BY WEIGHT

To convert ounces to grams, multiply the number of ounces by 30.

1 oz	¹⁄₁₆ lb	30 g
4 oz	¼ lb	120 g
8 oz	½ lb	240 g
12 oz	¾ lb	360 g
16 oz	1 lb	480 g

USEFUL EQUIVALENTS FOR COOKING/OVEN TEMPERATURES

Process	Fahrenheit	Celsius	Gas Mark
Freeze Water	32°F	0°C	
Room Temperature	68°F	20°C	
Boil Water	212°F	100°C	
Bake	325°F	160°C	3
	350°F	180°C	4
	375°F	190°C	5
	400°F	200°C	6
	425°F	220°C	7
	450°F	230°C	8
Broil			Grill

USEFUL EQUIVALENTS FOR LENGTH

To convert inches to centimeters, multiply the number of inches by 2.5.

1 in			2.5 cm	
6 in	½ ft		15 cm	
12 in	1 ft		30 cm	
36 in	3 ft	1 yd	90 cm	
40 in			100 cm	1 m

ENDNOTES

Chapter 1: The Hundred Trillion Friends You Didn't Know You Had

1. Andrew T. Stefka et al., "Commensal Bacteria Protect Against Food Allergen Sensitization," *Proceedings of the National Academy of Sciences* 111, no. 36 (September 9, 2014): 13145–13150: www.pnas.org /content/111/36/13145.

2. E. A. Huff, "People Who Eat Processed Junk Food Are Angry, Irritable, Say Scientists," *Natural News* (March 27, 2013): www.naturalnews.com/039655_processed_food_irritability_research.html.

3. N. Sudo et al., "Postnatal Microbial Colonization Programs the Hypothalamic–Pituitary–Adrenal System for Stress Response in Mice," *Journal of Physiology* 558, pt. 1 (July 2004): 263–275: abstract at http://www .ncbi.nlm.nih.gov/pubmed/15133062.

Chapter 2: The Trilogy

1. M. Roussin, *Analyses of Kombucha Ferments* (Fruita, Colorado: Information Resources, LC, 1996–2003): 25; kombucha-research.com.

2. D. Czerucka, T. Piche, and P. Rampal, "Review Article: Yeast as Probiotics—Saccharomyces boulardii," *Alimentary Pharmacology & Therapeutics* 26, no. 6 (September 15, 2007): 767–78: abstract at www.ncbi .nlm.nih.gov/pubmed/17767461.

3. C. H. Choi et al., "A Randomized, Double-Blind, Placebo-Controlled Multicenter Trial of Saccharomyces boulardii in Irritable Bowel Syndrome: Effect on Quality of Life," *Journal of Clinical Gastroenterology* 45, no. 8 (September 2011): 679–83: abstract at www.ncbi.nlm.nih.gov/pubmed/21301358; S. Uhlen, F. Toursel, and F. Gottrand, Association Française de Pédiatrie Ambulatoire, "Treatment of Acute Diarrhea: Prescription Patterns by Private Practice Pediatricians," *Archives de Pédiatrie* 11, no. 8 (August 2004): 903–7: abstract at http://www.ncbi.nlm.nih.gov/pubmed/15288079.

4. K. M. Cho et al., "Biodegradation of Chlorpyrifos by Lactic Acid Bacteria During Kimchi Fermentation," *Journal of Agricultural and Food Chemistry* 57, no. 5 (March 11, 2009): 1882–9: abstract at www.ncbi.nlm .nih.gov/pubmed/19199784.

5. "Cabbage Cure for Bird Flu?" FoodNavigator-Asia.com (March 16, 2005): www.foodnavigator-asia.com /Nutrition/Cabbage-cure-for-bird-flu.

Chapter 3: Prebiotics: Another Digestive Ally

1.   Jeff Leach, "(Re)Becoming Human," Human Food Project (September 30, 2014): humanfoodproject.com
     /rebecoming-human-happened-day-replaced-99-genes-body-hunter-gatherer.

Chapter 4: Your Health and Cultured Foods

1.   F. Indrio et al., "Prophylactic Use of a Probiotic in the Prevention of Colic, Regurgitation, and Functional
     Constipation: A Randomized Clinical Trial," *JAMA Pediatrics* 168, no. 3 (March 2014): 228–233:
     archpedi.jamanetwork.com/article.aspx?articleid=1812293.

2.   M. J. Blaser, *Missing Microbes: How the Overuse of Antibiotics Is Fueling Our Modern Plagues (New York: Henry
     Holt Publishing, 2014): 123-9.*

3.   J. Alcock, C. C. Maley, and C. A. Aktipis, "Is Eating Behavior Manipulated by the Gastrointestinal
     Microbiota? Evolutionary Pressures and Potential Mechanisms," *BioEssays* 36, no. 10 (October 2014):
     940–949:
     http://onlinelibrary.wiley.com/doi/10.1002/bies.201400071/full.

4.   C. Kresser, "RHR: Naturally Get Rid of Acne by Fixing Your Gut," ChrisKresser.com (December 21, 2011):
     chriskresser.com/naturally-get-rid-of-acne-by-fixing-your-gut.

5.   W. P. Bowe and A. C. Logan, "Acne Vulgaris, Probiotics and the Gut-Brain-Skin Axis—Back to the Future?"
     Gut Pathology 3, no. 1 (2011): www.ncbi.nlm.nih.gov/pmc/articles/PMC3038963.

6.   H. Zhang et al., "Risk Factors for Sebaceous Gland Diseases and Their Relationship to Gastrointestinal
     Dysfunction in Han Adolescents," *Journal of Dermatology* 35, no. 9 (September 2008): 555–61: abstract at
     www.ncbi.nlm.nih.gov/pubmed/18837699.

7.   C. Potera, "Asthma: A Gut Reaction to Antibiotics," *Environmental Health Perspectives* 113, no. 6 (June
     2005): A372: www.ncbi.nlm.nih.gov/pmc/articles/PMC1257633.

8.   K. Ivory et al., "Oral Delivery of Lactobacillus casei Shirota Modifies Allergen-Induced Immune Responses
     to Allergic Rhinitis," *Clinical & Experimental Allergy* 38, no. 8 (August 2008): 1282–9: abstract at www.ncbi
     .nlm.nih.gov/pubmed/18510694.

9.   "Adrenal Function in Allergies," AdrenalFatigue.org: www.adrenalfatigue.org/allergies.

10. K. R. Risnes et al., "Antibiotic Exposure by 6 Months and Asthma and Allergy at 6 Years: Findings in a
     Cohort of 1,401 US Children," *American Journal of Epidemiology* 173, no. 3 (February 1, 2011): 310–8: aje
     .oxfordjournals.org/content/173/3/310.full.

11. A. Semic-Jusufagic et al., "Assessing the Association of Early Life Antibiotic Prescription with Asthma
     Exacerbations, Impaired Antiviral Immunity, and Genetic Variants in 17q21: A Population-Based Birth
     Cohort Study," *The Lancet Respiratory Medicine* 2, no. 8 (August 2014): 621–30: www.thelancet.com
     /journals/lanres/article/PIIS2213-2600%2814%2970096-7/fulltext.

12. J. Scott and G. Gibson, "Probiotics and Autism," Food Matters (2007): www.foodsmatter.com/nutrition
     _micronutrition/pre_and_probiotics/articles/probiotics_and_autism.html.

13. J. A. Gilbert et al., "Toward Effective Probiotics for Autism and Other Neurodevelopmental Disorders," *Cell* 155, no. 7 (December 19, 2013): 1446–8: www.sciencedirect.com/science/article/pii /S0092867413014864.

14. D. Patton, "Sauerkraut Consumption May Fight Off Breast Cancer," NUTRAIngredients (November 4, 2005): www.nutraingredients.com/Research/Sauerkraut-consumption-may-fight-off-breast-cancer.

15. H. Szaefer et al., "Modulation of CYP1A1, CYP1A2 and CYP1B1 Expression by Cabbage Juices and Indoles in Human Breast Cell Lines," *Nutrition and Cancer* 64, no. 6 (August 2012): 879–88: abstract at www.ncbi .nlm.nih.gov/pubmed/22716309.

16. A. Grishina et al., "Antigenotoxic Effect of Kefir and Ayran Supernatants on Fecal Water-Induced DNA Damage in Human Colon Cells," *Nutrition and Cancer* 63, no. 1 (2011): 73–9: abstract at www.ncbi.nlm .nih.gov/pubmed/21161824

17. J. Gao et al., "Induction of Apoptosis of Gastric Cancer Cells SGC7901 In Vitro by a Cell-Free Fraction of Tibetan Kefir," *International Dairy Journal* 30, no. 1 (May 2013): 14–18: www.sciencedirect.com/science /article/pii/S0958694612002658.

18. A. de Moreno de Leblanc et al., "Study of Immune Cells Involved in the Antitumor Effect of Kefir in a Murine Breast Cancer Model," *Journal of Dairy Science* 90, no. 4 (April 2007):1920–8: www .journalofdairyscience.org/article/S0022-0302%2807%2971678-8/fulltext.

19. L. G. van der Flier and H. Clevers, "Stem Cells, Self Renewal, and Differentiation in the Intestinal Epithelium," *Annual Review of Physiology* 71, (2009): 241–60: abstract at science.naturalnews. com/2009/2043215_Stem_cells_self_renewal_and_differentiation_in_the_intestinal_epithelium.html; L. Bailey, "Gut Reaction: Mice Survive Lethal Doses of Chemotherapy," *Michigan News* (July 31, 2013): ns.umich.edu/new/releases/21613-digest-this-cure-for-cancer-may-live-in-our-intestines.

20. WebMD, "Find a Vitamin or Supplement: Lactobacillus": www.webmd.com/vitamins-supplements/ ingredientmono-790-lactobacillus.aspx?activeIngredientId=790&activeIngredientName=lactobacillus&source=1.

21. "Brothers in Arms: Commensal Bacteria Help Fight Viruses, According to Penn Study," *Penn Medicine* (June 18, 2012): www.uphs.upenn.edu/news/News_Releases/2012/06/brothers.

22. R. Bibiloni et al., "VSL#3 Probiotic-Mixture Induces Remission in Patients with Active Ulcerative Colitis," *American Journal of Gastroenterology* 100, no. 7 (July 2005): 1539–46: abstract at www.ncbi.nlm.nih.gov /pubmed/15984978.

23. A. Tursi et al., "Treatment of Relapsing Mild-to-Moderate Ulcerative Colitis with the Probiotic VSL # 3 as Adjunctive to a Standard Pharmaceutical Treatment: A Double-Blind, Randomized, Placebo-Controlled Study," *American Journal of Gastroenterology* 105, no. 10 (October 2010): 2218–87: www.med.upenn.edu /gastro/documents/VSL3Tursi.pdf.

24. "Study Reveals That People May Inherit 'Gut' Bacteria That Cause Crohn's Disease and Ulcerative Colitis," University of Minnesota *Discover: Science + Technology* (December 16, 2014): discover.umn.edu/news /science-technology/people-may-inherit-gut-bacteria-cause-crohns-disease-and-ulcerative-colitis.

25. N. Borruel et al., "Increased Mucosal Tumor Necrosis Factor α Production in Crohn's Disease Can Be Downregulated Ex Vivo By Probiotic Bacteria," *Gut* 51, no. 5 (2002): 659–64: gut.bmj.com /content/51/5/659.full.

26. A. Hadhazy, "Think Twice: How the Gut's 'Second Brain' Influences Mood and Well-Being," *Scientific American Online* (February 12, 2010): www.scientificamerican.com/article/gut-second-brain.

27. S. Carpenter, "That Gut Feeling," *Monitor on Psychology* 43, no. 8 (September 2012): 50: www.apa.org /monitor/2012/09/gut-feeling.aspx.

28. A. C. Bested, A. C. Logan, and E. M Selhub, "Intestinal Microbiota, Probiotics and Mental Health: From Metchnikoff to Modern Advances. Part III—Convergence Toward Clinical Trials," *Gut Pathogens* 5, no. 1 (March 16, 2013): 4: www.ncbi.nlm.nih.gov/pmc/articles/PMC3605358.

29. L. Desbonnet et al., "The Probiotic Bifidobacteria infantis: An Assessment of Potential Antidepressant Properties in the Rat," *Journal of Psychiatric Research* 43, no. 2 (December 2008): 164–74: abstract at www .ncbi.nlm.nih.gov/pubmed/18456279; R. Wall et al., "Impact of Administered Bifidobacterium on Murine Host Fatty Acid Composition," *Lipids* 45, no. 5 (May 2010):429–36: abstract at www.ncbi.nlm.nih.gov /pubmed/20405232.

30. B. Watson with L. Smith, M. D., *The Skinny Gut Diet: Balance Your Digestive System for Permanent Weight Loss* (New York: Harmony Books, 2014): x–xiii.

31. A. Everard et al., "Cross-Talk Between *Akkermansia muciniphila* and Intestinal Epithelium Controls Diet-Induced Obesity," *Proceedings of the National Academy of Sciences* 110, no. 22 (May 28, 2013): 9066–71: www.pnas.org/content/110/22/9066.full.

32. G. Triadafilopoulos, R. W. Simms, and D. L. Goldenberg, "Bowel Dysfunction in Fibromyalgia Syndrome," *Digestive Diseases and Sciences* 36, no. 1 (January 1991): 59–64: abstract at www.ncbi.nlm.nih.gov /pubmed/1985007.

33. D. J. Wallace and D. S. Hallegua, "Fibromyalgia: The Gastrointestinal Link," *Current Pain and Headache Reports* 8, no. 5 (October 2004): 364–8: abstract at www.ncbi.nlm.nih.gov/pubmed/15361320.

34. C. Kresser, "Is Fibromyalgia Caused by SIBO and Leaky Gut?" ChrisKresser.com (June 6, 2014): chriskresser .com/is-fibromyalgia-caused-by-sibo-and-leaky-gut.

35. "Food Allergy, or Something Else?" WebMD: www.webmd.com/allergies/foods-allergy-intolerance.

36. A. T. Stefka, et al., "Commensal Bacteria Protect Against Food Allergen Sensitization," *Proceedings of the National Academy of Sciences* 111, no. 36 (September 9, 2014): 13145–13150: www.pnas.org /content/111/36/13145.

37. J. Mercola, "Higher Levels of Magnesium Linked with Lower Heart Attack Rate," Mercola.com (December 16, 2010): articles.mercola.com/sites/articles/archive/2010/12/16/higher-levels-of-this-mineral-linked -with-lower-heart-attack-rate.aspx.

38. S. C. Larsson, N. Orsini, and A. Wolk, "Dietary Magnesium Intake and Risk of Stroke: A Meta-Analysis of Prospective Studies," *American Journal of Clinical Nutrition* 95, no. 2 (February 2012): 362–6: http://ajcn .nutrition.org/content/95/2/362.full.pdf+html.

39. Y. Hata et al., "A Placebo-Controlled Study of the Effect of Sour Milk on Blood Pressure in Hypertensive Subjects," *American Journal of Clinical Nutrition* 64, no. 5 (November 1996): 767–71: ajcn.nutrition.org /content/64/5/767.full.pdf.

40. J. Y. Dong et al., "Effect of Probiotic Fermented Milk on Blood Pressure: A Meta-Analysis of Randomised Controlled Trials," *British Journal of Nutrition* 110, no. 7 (October 2013): 1188–1194: abstract at www.ncbi .nlm.nih.gov/pubmed/23823502.

41. M. C. Fuentes et al., "Cholesterol-Lowering Efficacy of Lactobacillus plantarum CECT 7527, 7528 and 7529 in Hypercholesterolaemic Adults," *British Journal of Nutrition* 109, no. 10 (May 28, 2013): 1866–72: abstract at www.ncbi.nlm.nih.gov/pubmed/23017585.

42. M. L. Jones et al., "Cholesterol-Lowering Efficacy of a Microencapsulated Bile Salt Hydrolase-Active Lactobacillus reuteri NCIMB 30242 Yoghurt Formulation in Hypercholesterolaemic Adults," *British Journal of Nutrition* 107, no. 10 (May 2012): 1505–13: abstract at www.ncbi.nlm.nih.gov/pubmed/22067612.

43. B. Keating, "New Dairy Product Fights Cholesterol," Online Ag at OSU, a Division of Agricultural Sciences and Natural Resources/Oklahoma State University: www.okstate.edu/ag/agedcm4h/ag_news/ag@osu /fa96/afa96_4.htm.

44. "Impact of Gut Microbiota of Fermented Milk Product Containing Probiotics Revealed by New Technology," *Science Daily* (September 11, 2014): www.sciencedaily.com /releases/2014/09/140911125045.htm.

45. A. Agrawal et al., "Clinical Trial: The Effects of a Fermented Milk Product Containing Bifidobacterium lactis DN-173 010 on Abdominal Distension and Gastrointestinal Transit in Irritable Bowel Syndrome with Constipation," *Alimentary Pharmacology and Therapeutics* 29, no. 1 (January 2009): 104–14: abstract at www.ncbi.nlm.nih.gov/pubmed/18801055.

46. H. Østgaard et al., "Diet and Effects of Diet Management on Quality of Life and Symptoms in Patients with Irritable Bowel Syndrome," *Molecular Medicine Reports* 5, no. 6 (June 2012): 1382–90: www.spandidos -publications.com/10.3892/mmr.2012.843.

47. N. Ranganathan et al., "Pilot Study of Probiotic Dietary Supplementation for Promoting Healthy Kidney Function in Patients with Chronic Kidney Disease," *Advances in Therapy* 27, no. 9 (September 2010): 634– 47: www.academia.edu/2108877/Pilot_Study_of_Probiotic_Dietary_Supplementation_for_Promoting _Healthy_Kidney_Function_in_Patients_with_Chronic_Kidney_Disease.

48. S. Duncan et al., "Oxalobacter formigenes and Its Potential Role in Human Health," *Applied and Environmental Microbiology* 68, no. 8 (August 2002): 3841–7: aem.asm.org/content/68/8/3841.full.

49. C. Campieri et al., "Reduction of Oxaluria after an Oral Course of Lactic Acid Bacteria at High Concentration," *Kidney International* 60, no. 3 (September 2001): 1097–105: abstract at www.ncbi.nlm .nih.gov/pubmed/11532105.

50. J. C. Lieskie et al., "Use of a Probiotic to Decrease Enteric Hyperoxaluria," *Kidney International* 68, no. 3 (September 2005): 1244–9: abstract at www.ncbi.nlm.nih.gov/pubmed/16105057.

51. R. Kellman, *The Microbiome Diet: The Scientifically Proven Way to Restore Your Gut Health and Achieve Permanent Weight Loss,* Boston, Da Capo Press (2014): product description.

52. D. Lesbros-Pantoflickova, I. Corthésy-Theulaz, and A. L. Blum, "Helicobacter pylori and Probiotics," *Journal of Nutrition* 137, no. 3 (March 2007): 812S–85: jn.nutrition.org/content/137/3/812S.full.

53. S. Elmståhl, U. Svensson, and G. Berglund, "Fermented Milk Products Are Associated to Ulcer Disease. Results from a Cross-Sectional Population Study," *European Journal of Clinical Nutrition* 52, no. 9 (September 1998): 668–74: abstract at www.ncbi.nlm.nih.gov/pubmed/9756124.

54. W. H. Aldoori et al., "Prospective Study of Diet and the Risk of Duodenal Ulcer in Men," *American Journal of Epidemiology* 145, no. 1 (1997): 42–50: aje.oxfordjournals.org/content/145/1/42.full.pdf.

55. D. Banerjee et al., "Comparative Healing Property of Kombucha Tea and Black Tea Against Indomethacin-Induced Gastric Ulceration in Mice: Possible Mechanism of Action," *Food & Function* 1, no. 3 (December 2010): 284–93: abstract at www.ncbi.nlm.nih.gov/pubmed/21776478.

56. G. Cheney, S. H. Waxler, and I. J. Miller, "Vitamin U Therapy of Peptic Ulcer; Experience at San Quentin Prison," *California Medicine* 84, no. 1 (January 1956): 39–42: abstract at www.ncbi.nlm.nih.gov/pubmed/13276831; G. Cheney, "Rapid Healing of Peptic Ulcers in Patients Receiving Fresh Cabbage Juice," *California Medicine* 70, no. 1 (January 1949): 10–15: abstract at www.ncbi.nlm.nih.gov/pubmed/18104715.

57. S. Kumar et al., "Evaluation of Efficacy of Probiotics in Prevention of Candida Colonization in PICU: A Randomized Controlled Trial," *Critical Care Medicine* 41, no. 2 (February 2013): 565–72: abstract at www.ncbi.nlm.nih.gov/pubmed/23361033.

58. R. C. Martinez et al., "Effect of Lactobacillus rhamnosus GR-1 and Lactobacillus reuteri RC-14 on the Ability of Candida albicans to Infect Cells and Induce Inflammation," *Microbiology and Immunology* 53, no. 9 (September 2009): 487–95: abstract at www.ncbi.nlm.nih.gov/pubmed/19703242; K.C. Anukam et al., "Clinical Study Comparing Probiotic Lactobacillus GR-1 and RC-14 with Metronidazole Vaginal Gel to Treat Symptomatic Bacterial Vaginosis," *Microbes and Infection* 8, nos. 12–13 (October 2006): 2772–6: abstract at www.ncbi.nlm.nih.gov/pubmed/17045832.

INDEX

ACKNOWLEDGMENTS

"If you hang out with chickens, you're going to cluck,
and if you hang out with eagles, you're going to fly."
—Steve Maraboli

As I finish up the final touches on my book, I feel an ocean of gratitude. I once again completely understand the saying "Success feels so much better when it is shared." This is how I feel about the people in my life who helped me accomplish the task of completing this book. There have been so many times when I felt my shortcomings, but each time I did the right person showed up in my life to teach me and give me encouragement. I hope this book and my life will be a blessing to others just as the people in this section are a blessing to me. We are all brothers and sisters who help each other with our special talents and gifts. This is what makes life so magical!

To my mom and dad, who always loved and supported me and encouraged me to follow my heart. Mom, thank you for letting me talk endlessly about all I'm doing. Although the busyness has made the phone calls fewer, you're always there just when I need to hear your voice. I love you so much. To my dad, who resides in the heavens above, it still feels like you're right beside me, laughing and telling me, "You're pretty terrific." Death cannot separate those who love one another, and I can still feel your presence in my life.

To my husband, Ron, after 31 years of marriage I can honestly say you are the most unselfish and giving person I have ever met. There would be no books or Cultured Food Life if I didn't have your strength and example of how to run your own business. I still laugh every time you wink at me and say, "Remember I was your initial investor." But it wasn't just the support you gave me financially to start my business; it was your strong character and your vast love. Thank you for taking on the enormous task of building me a store and for shipping literally 3.3 tons of products last year! Thank you for never tiring of trying my many recipes and for being there when I need your big, broad shoulders to lift me up so I can soar even higher. Life with you is an adventure, and we have a special love story that has stood the test of time. Love you.

To my editor, Laura, people underestimate how much an editor contributes to helping an author create a book. You persuaded me to add to this book in ways I never imagined. You brought out the best in me and allowed me to learn things I otherwise would have missed. I loved living in the little world that we created while making *CFFH*. It felt like a creative haven that was filled with hard work, laughter, and so much fun! Thank you for putting not only your expertise but your heart into my book. When it gets into the hands of readers, they will feel your essence alongside mine. Thank you for being my editor, friend, and mentor. You're a treasure to me.

To my daughter Maci, thank you for the pictures that make my book so beautiful. Thank you for being the first person I call when I need a pickup. You have surprised me again and again, and I love that my own flesh and blood makes me strive to be better in word, thought, and deed. I am so proud of you and consider you one of my very best friends. I miss you terribly since you moved to sunny California, but having you be a part of my team has eased the burden. And it gives me hope that we will be together again someday.

To my daughter Holli, I shall always remember this summer as a magical time. It was special because I spent it with you while writing my book. Writing by day and watching Harry Potter movies by night made for a mystical world that only you and I lived in. Walking barefoot on the ground and pretending we could accomplish anything made me feel like I could soar. Holli, you're the one who spends the most time with me, and your gentle spirit is the sweetest force that keeps me grounded and looking for magic . . . *in the woods.*

To my son, D.J., you inspire me every time I'm around you. I remember after I finished my first book, you looked at me and said, "What's the next thing you want to do? Don't you need another challenge?" Thank you for all the late-night deep and meaningful talks. I can't wait to see what you do next. Don't *you* want another challenge? I'm waiting to see what you'll do next!

To Chris Johnston, thank you not only for making all my websites beautiful and keeping everything running smoothly but also for being creative, inspiring, and steady. We have fun in this process of creation, and there is so much more to come. I see greatness in you and always have. I count it as a gift to have you in my life and business. I am sorry for the millions of text messages and hundreds of problems that a business creates, but you lift the pressure again and again. Together we have done the impossible and this has made us mighty!

To Jane Horning, who has made me a better writer by editing all my blogs and taking so much pressure off me. You've been a welcome addition to not only my business but also my life. I love how you share your heart with me and how I feel so comfortable sharing mine with you. I hope we will have many more years of fun and growth together.

To Jennifer England, thank you for all the editing, especially your expertise in scientific footnotes. I really enjoy working with you and hope to do much more of it in the future. Thanks for always supporting me and being someone I so enjoy talking to. You have so many gifts and talents that so many have yet to discover. I hope you will use them and enrich us all.

To Jeremiah England, who is the best videographer a girl could have. We have created such wonderful things together, and I hope to do so much more. You're an inspiration to watch and probably one of the most creative people I have ever known. I get a thrill each time you move to higher and higher levels of success. You're doing exactly what you should be doing—and you're doing a fabulous job!

To Shelley Hanna, who has done more for me than just make graphics and fabulous recipes. I appreciate your support again and again throughout this whole process of writing a book. Few people know of how you have influenced my life just by being you. Your friendship, long talks, and help at my classes mean the world to me. There is nothing better than having Shelley there. I have reserved a special place in my family just for you.

To my sister Danette, who lets me call her when I don't know how to interpret scientific data and then makes sense of it all. Thank you for encouraging me to write a book, listening to all my dilemmas, and helping me go for my dreams. I have always been proud of your success in business and your Ph.D. in science. You make me believe that I can do something special, too, for after all, we have the same genes.

To all my sisters, Diane, Debbie, and Danette, who have supported me, even when I've been too busy. It's your friendship and how hard we laugh together that I love the most. You make me realize how lucky I am to have such a wonderful family.

To Patty Gift, thank you for believing in me and for radiating warmth and kindness in all you do. I've never met anyone who aspires to such excellence in thought and deed and then inspires the same in me. Working and knowing you has enriched my life. When I grow up, I want to be just like you.

To the fabulous staff at Hay House: Reid, Margarete, Dani, Darcy, Erin, Marlene, Sally, Richelle, and so many more. I'm grateful for all your wisdom and expertise. What a privilege to be a part of the Hay House family, which is a direct reflection of all of you. I have yet to meet one person from Hay House who is not warm, kind, and great at her job! Thank you for all you do. I am most grateful.

ABOUT THE AUTHOR

Donna Schwenk is the author of *Cultured Food for Life* and the founder of www .culturedfoodlife.com. For a decade she was the Kansas City chapter leader for the Weston A. Price Foundation, a worldwide organization made up of people dedicated to restoring nutrient-dense food to the human diet through education, research, and activism. Donna teaches classes around the country to open people's eyes to the power of cultured foods, which dramatically changed her health and the health of her family when she began making and eating them in 2002. She and her work have been featured on radio and television—including two PBS specials—in Britain's *Daily Mail,* and in magazines including *Energy Times, Vegetarian Times,* and *Mother Earth News.*

NOTES

Hay House Titles of Related Interest

YOU CAN HEAL YOUR LIFE, the movie, starring Louise Hay & Friends
(available as an online streaming video)
www.hayhouse.com/louise-movie

THE SHIFT, the movie, starring Dr. Wayne W. Dyer
(available as an online streaming video)
www.hayhouse.com/the-shift-movie

✸

*CRAZY SEXY JUICE: 100+ Simple Juice, Smoothie & Nut Milk Recipes
to Supercharge Your Health,* by Kris Carr

THE EARTH DIET: Your Complete Guide to Living Using Earth's Natural Ingredients,
by Liana Werner-Gray

LOVING YOURSELF TO GREAT HEALTH: Thoughts & Food—the Ultimate Diet,
by Louise Hay, Ahlea Khadro, and Heather Dane

MAKE YOUR OWN RULES DIET,
by Tara Stiles

THE MYSTIC COOKBOOK: The Secret Alchemy of Food,
by Denise Linn and Meadow Linn

All of the above are available at your local bookstore,
or may be ordered by contacting Hay House (see next page).

✸

We hope you enjoyed this Hay House book. If you'd like to receive
our online catalog featuring additional information on Hay House
books and products, or if you'd like to find out more about the
Hay Foundation, please contact:

Hay House, Inc., P.O. Box 5100, Carlsbad, CA 92018-5100
(760) 431-7695 or (800) 654-5126
(760) 431-6948 (fax) or (800) 650-5115 (fax)
www.hayhouse.com® • www.hayfoundation.org

———

Published in Australia by: Hay House Australia Pty. Ltd.,
18/36 Ralph St., Alexandria NSW 2015
Phone: 612-9669-4299 • *Fax:* 612-9669-4144
www.hayhouse.com.au

Published in the United Kingdom by: Hay House UK, Ltd.,
The Sixth Floor, Watson House, 54 Baker Street, London W1U 7BU
Phone: +44 (0)20 3927 7290 • *Fax:* +44 (0)20 3927 7291
www.hayhouse.co.uk

Published in India by: Hay House Publishers India,
Muskaan Complex, Plot No. 3, B-2, Vasant Kunj, New Delhi 110 070
Phone: 91-11-4176-1620 • *Fax:* 91-11-4176-1630
www.hayhouse.co.in

———

Access New Knowledge.
Anytime. Anywhere.

Learn and evolve at your own pace
with the world's leading experts.

www.hayhouseU.com

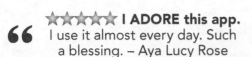

Printed in the United States
by Baker & Taylor Publisher Services